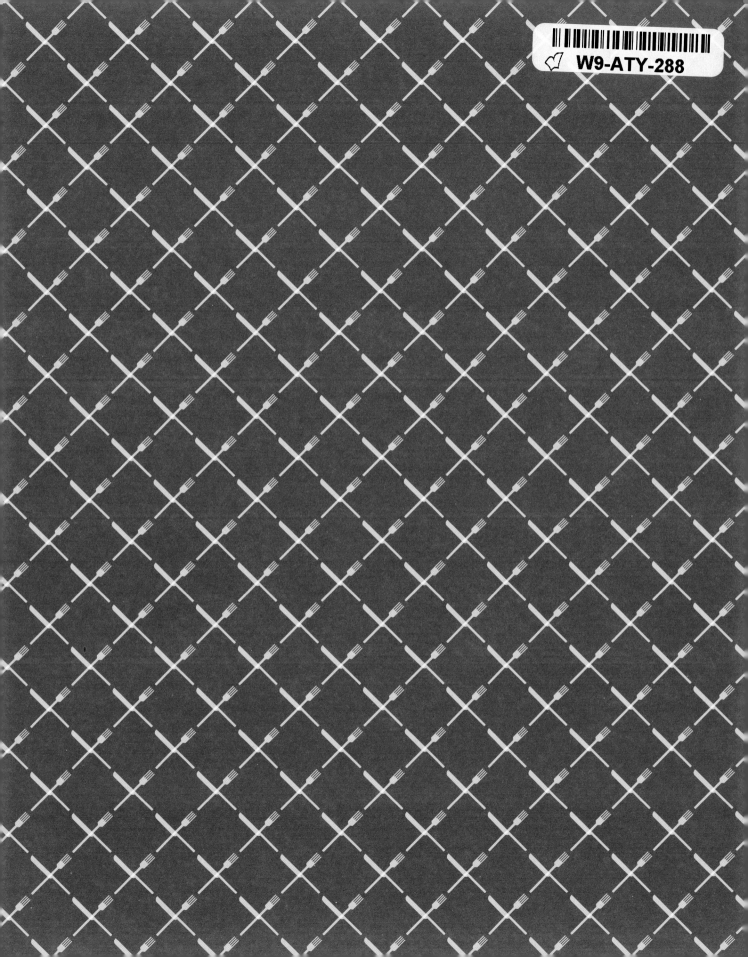

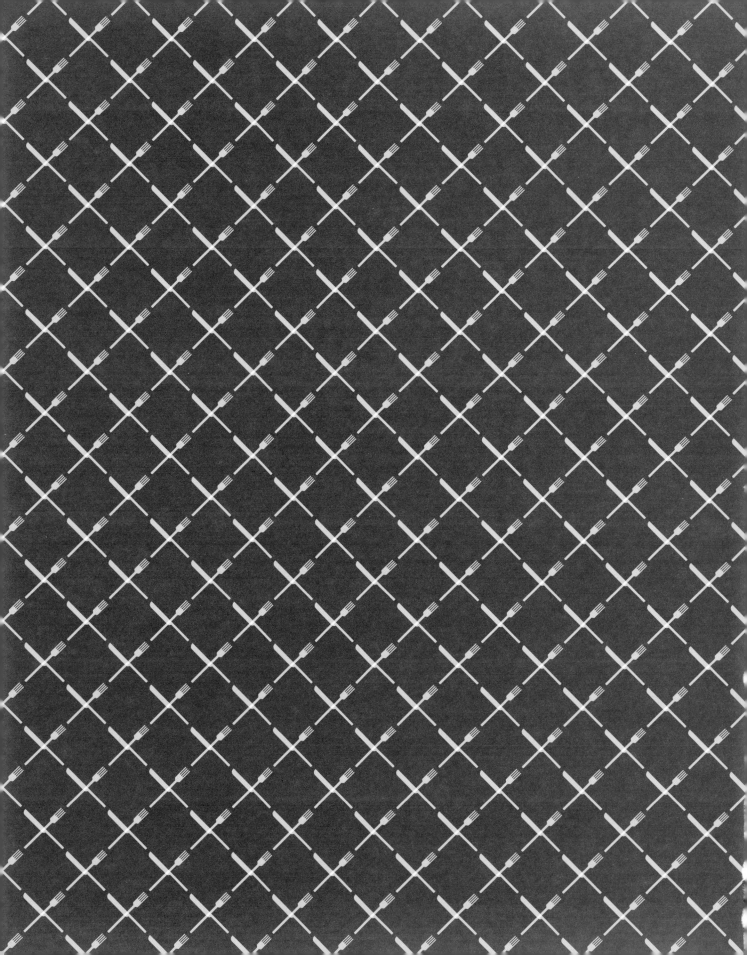

KETOGENTIC DIET
COOKBOOK

OVER 100 RECIPES

TO IMPROVE YOUR HEALTH, FROM WEIGHT LOSS
AND BLOOD SUGAR CONTROL, TO RENEWED ENERGY
AND BETTER MENTAL FOCUS!

EDITED BY

SAHIL MAKHIJA

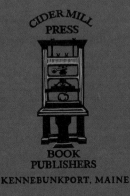

CIDER MILL PRESS

BOOK
PUBLISHERS
KENNEBUNKPORT, MAINE

The Ketogenic Diet Cookbook
Copyright © 2018 by Appleseed Press Book Publishers LLC.

This is an officially licensed book by Cider Mill Press Book Publishers LLC.

13-Digit ISBN: 978-1604337945
10-Digit ISBN: 160433794X

This book may be ordered by mail from the publisher. Please include $5.99 for postage and handling. Please support your local bookseller first!

Books published by Cider Mill Press Book Publishers are available at special discounts for bulk purchases in the United States by corporations, institutions, and other organizations. For more information, please contact the publisher.

Cider Mill Press Book Publishers
"Where good books are ready for press"
PO Box 454
12 Spring Street
Kennebunkport, Maine 04046
Visit us online!
cidermillpress.com

Design by Cindy Butler
Typography: Eveleth, Avenir Next
Image Credits: All images used under official license from Shutterstock.com.

Printed in China
1 2 3 4 5 6 7 8 9 0
First Edition

CONTENTS

INTRODUCTION

Is there a more dismal word in the English language than "diet"? Somewhere in the 20th century, it lost its meaning as "the normal course of food consumed by a person" and instead became associated with restriction, deprivation, and sacrifice in the hopes of achieving a health goal. Diet became a sad word, as did the pursuit of health.

No more. We're here to reclaim the word. What if we told you you could lose weight and become healthier by eating bacon and cheese? And butter. And all the steaks you want. Does that sound like a diet?

This is the ketogenic diet—keto, for short—which is a high-fat, adequate-protein, low-carb way of eating. It turns your body into a fat-burning machine, fine-tuning your metabolism to burn your body's years of stored-up fat. What this does is reset your understanding of food, and help you use what you eat to improve your energy levels and mood, regulate hormones, stabilize your blood sugar levels, enhance you mental clarity… and lose weight, of course. But weight loss is only one of its many incidental benefits.

UNLEARN EVERYTHING

For decades now, we've been told that fat is bad, that saturated fats are responsible for raising cholesterol and bringing on heart disease, which had become a sort of epidemic in America by the 1970s. The "diet-heart hypothesis," introduced in the 1980s, linked fat to bad health based on a few animal studies (none of which were carried out on humans) and passed into public policy even before research was complete and before the studies had drawn any solid conclusions. The result? Fat became the enemy. Butter was replaced by margarine. Red meat was off the

table and replaced by poultry, without skin, because that's where all the bad saturated fats hid. Full fat milk and milk products gave way to watery skim milk. Granola became a buzzword. A new health fad had begun—low-fat everything.

Yet, heart disease continued, unabated; as of this year, one in three deaths is attributed to cardiovascular disease in the US. Diabetes has skyrocketed, from 2.39 million people diagnosed in 1965 to 23.35 million people in 2015, without about 7 million more undiagnosed cases. Something was clearly wrong.

In the meantime, nutrition research has caught up. More and more medical studies have disproved the role of fat in heart disease and cholesterol. Long-term reviews found little difference in longevity between people over 60 with high and low LDL cholesterol. Focus has, instead, shifted to the role of processed carbs and sugar in our diet, both of which feature abundantly in the so-called health food being peddled by brands everywhere. It turns out we were looking at the wrong bad guy all this time.

So fat, then, is our friend. Why? Fat is more energy-dense than carbohydrates—gram for gram, fat has more calories than carbs (9 calories per gram as opposed to 4 calories per gram of carbs). Carbs are broken down more quickly, finding its way into your system quicker, while fats burn slower and more level over a longer period, giving you a more stable source of energy. When you eat refined carbs and sugars, its super-quick breakdown spikes your insulin, causing a sharp rise and, subsequently, a crash in your energy levels. This yo-yoing of energy leaves you feeling drained and fatigued. Cut out carbs, and your body turns to its own fat for energy, which is the whole point of the keto diet. But it can take significant unlearning to learn to love fats after being conditioned to believe that they're bad for you. How do you get there faster? By cooking and eating tasty, healthy, high-fat food that will make you feel at your optimum. That is the essence of what this book is all about.

LIFESTYLE, NOT DIET

The key to embracing the keto way of eating is to think of it as a lifestyle and not a diet. While you are cutting out grains, sugars, and processed carbs, you're not cutting out food. Instead, you're encouraged to your fill and eat well. How could you possibly feel like you're on a restricted diet when you're tucking into scrambled eggs (page 14), bouillabaisse (page 43), buffalo wings (page 75), or a porterhouse steak (page 121)? The recipes in this book span the spectrum from familiar comfort food, to family favorites, to party nibbles and, of course, indulgences to treat yourself with. Are people telling you you can't eat dessert on keto? We've got 10 decadent dessert recipes to prove them wrong. What's more, each recipe comes with exact serving sizes and macros, so you can take the guesswork out of equation and focus on the important bit—enjoying the food.

And that's the other great thing about the ketogenic diet: so long as you're getting your fix of fats and proteins, you'll never be hungry. Hunger is the biggest hurdle in any diet, and most of them that focus on restricting calories or food intake leave you feeling dissatisfied and, consequently, "hangry." Hunger can also make you go off your diet a lot faster. Not on keto. Proteins and fats are the components of food that keep you sated longer, so not only are you not reaching for diet-breaking snacks, but you're also not turning into the angry Hulk between meals.

So, then, is keto all about eating bacon and butter at every meal? Not at all. Keto is all about eating real food: good fats, healthy proteins and carbs derived from fresh greens and veggies. Don't fear the carbs in vegetables; most above-ground vegetables have fairly low glycemic indices that won't trigger an insulin spike. You want to avoid root vegetables and tubers like potatoes and beetroot—by nature they're full of starches that the plant needs to grow, which are not keto-conducive. A lot of keto dieters will tell you that you can't eat more than 20 grams of carbs; this is not always true. Everyone has a different carb tolerance and while some people can eat up to 50 grams of carbs and stay in ketosis, some will get kicked out if they go over 30 grams. The trick is to find your sweet spot.

The truth, though, is that keto doesn't need the overthinking. It's easy and, trust us, it's the most enjoyable way of eating you'll ever have tried. When you're feeling as good as you do on keto, it stops becoming that dreaded word—diet—and instead becomes a lifestyle you'll want to sustain for life. So ditch those carbs and make friends with fat, and enjoy the journey to great health on keto. We're here to help.

The ketogenic diet goes by many names—low-carb, low carb high fat (LCHF), keto—but at the heart of it the concept remains the same: deprive your body of carbs,so it can turn to fat and stored body fat for energy through a process called "ketosis."

WHAT IS KETOSIS?

Normally, our bodies use glucose as a primary source of energy, derived through the carbohydrates we eat. On the keto diet, we deprive our body of these carbs by limiting our consumption of them to under 20-30 grams in a day, or, to roughly 5% of our total intake of food. When this happens, our body has to find an alternate source of fuel to keep us going, and that is where ketosis kicks in, where our body starts to use fat for energy. The liver converts fatty acids into ketone bodies that the brain and other organs can use as fuel.

WHAT'S SO GREAT ABOUT KETO?

Well, for starters, keto effectively turns your body into a fat burning machine, making it a great way to lose weight, while also lowering your overall body fat. But you don't need to have a weight problem to be following the keto diet—a lot of people find that it gives them greater mental clarity, lowers cholesterol and blood pressure, and keeps them away from processed and sugar-heavy food that has now shown to be the cause many lifestyle diseases.

When you eat high fat and moderate protein, you will also find that you are far more satiated and satisfied with you meals. Not craving those in-between-meals snacks is half the battle won!

The keto diet has also been known to be very effective in helping people who suffer from diabetes, epilepsy, and a number of other autoimmune diseases. In fact, the diet is not new; it was actually formulated for epilepsy patients and was found to greatly reduce the frequency and intensity of seizures. We're only now realizing the many other benefits that come from following the keto lifestyle.

WHAT, EXACTLY, IS THE ROLE OF INSULIN IN KETO?

If you've been eating carbs, you're probably familiar with the post lunch slump, that hour or two when your energy dips after you eat rice, bread, or pasta for lunch (in other words, nap time!). That is a function of insulin—regulating the metabolism of carbohydrates and fats. After a carb-heavy meal, your pancreas produces insulin to help break down the glucose in it and convert it into glycogen that your body can use for energy. The insulin also triggers the production of serotonin and melatonin, which calm you down and induce sleep.

But insulin is also the hormone that converts excess glycogen to body fat, when your body has more carbs than it needs. When you eat carb- and sugar-heavy foods meal after meal, your insulin levels remain high for extended periods of time. Eventually, over time, your cells are unable to use the insulin effectively, leading to insulin resistance, which has been implicated in the rise of type 2 diabetes and many other autoimmune diseases.

On keto, with your carb levels so low, your glucose levels aren't elevated, and your insulin doesn't spike after a meal. Lower insulin levels means greater insulin sensitivity, cutting down on metabolic disorders and more effective fat burning. As a plus, you'll find you have greater mental clarity and a more stable level of energy throughout the day.

WHAT ARE MACROS AND WHY DO THEY MATTER?

Macros is short for macronutrients, which is the breakup of the components of your food. These include carbohydrates, proteins and fats—the three components that you should keep track of on keto. Macros can be tracked through fitness apps like MyFitnessPal or Lose It.

On a keto diet, it's important to monitor your daily macros, to ensure you're getting enough fat and just enough carbs. Ideally you could look at 70-75% of your daily calories coming from fat sources, 20-25% from protein, and 5-10% from carbohydrates, specifically net carbs. This is what will keep your body in ketosis and fat-burning mode.

WHAT ARE NET CARBS?

Most foods containing carbs have a dietary fiber or roughage component. Fiber is important for the body, because it helps with the absorption of nutrients in your gut and regulates bowel movements. A lot of dietary fiber is also insoluble and passes through your gut without being digested, so it doesn't count towards your total carb intake. Simply put, net carbs are the total amount of carbs in your food, minus the fiber. On keto, you want to keep you net carb intake to 5-10%.

WHAT KIND OF CARBOHYDRATES SHOULD MY 5-10% COMPRISE OF?

When it comes to consuming carbs on the keto diet, you want those to come largely from vegetables, specifically green leafy vegetables like spinach, kale, lettuce, chard, etc. Cruciferous vegetables like cauliflower and broccoli are high in fiber, and zucchini and eggplant are also good sources for those carbs. You want to avoid starchy veggies like potato, sweet potato, and corn—these are likely to kick you out of ketosis with just a mouthful. More colorful veggies like peppers, tomatoes, and red onions can be consumed, but they're best eaten in moderation. It's also possible that some of your carbs might come from dairy products like cheese, so you want to read those labels carefully. All grains and grain products are off the table. You want to be especially careful with storebought sauces and even mayonnaise; it's amazing how many hidden carbs they can have.

SO WHAT SHOULD I BE EATING ON KETO ?

Apart from the vegetables mentioned earlier, there is a whole lot to eat on the keto diet. When it comes to protein sources, you can pretty much eat all kinds of meat. This includes poultry like chicken, duck, turkey, and quail; red meats like beef, lamb, pork, and venison; and also eggs of all kinds. High fat dairy products like cream, cheese, butter, and full fat yogurt (in moderation) are all keto friendly, though you would want to avoid milk itself as its carb count is high. Nuts are a great source of good fats, especially macadamia nuts, hazelnuts, almonds, and walnuts but you want to be careful about eating peanuts and carb-heavy cashews in large quantities. This is why tracking macros are important, so you can keep a count on your overall carb intake.

Now, since sugar is completely off the table on keto, it eliminates most fruits from the diet. However, there are a few that fall into the keto-friendly category—mainly avocado and berries such as strawberries, raspberries, and blackberries. Once again, it's important to consume these in moderation in keeping with your macros.

Fats, the largest component of your diet, can come from both plant and animal sources. When choosing meat, choose fattier cuts, and eat poultry with the skin on, since that's where a lot of the fat is. The other sources of pure fat are your oils, healthy ones like olive, coconut, and avocado, besides ghee and butter. Animal fats like lard, bacon grease, and duck fat are not only healthy, but also add some serious flavor to all your food.

HOW DO I KNOW THAT I'M IN KETOSIS?

Ketosis is the state your body is in when it switches from a carb burning to a fat burning mechanism. In this state, your liver is actively converting fats into ketones, and these can be detected by the use of ketone detection strips. These strips measure the amount of ketones you excrete, though it's not always accurate. There are also blood ketone monitors and breath monitors, both of which are expensive and, frankly, unnecessary. The most important thing to do is to listen to your body, focus on the food and the nutrition you're getting.

There are also some symptoms that mark the transition into ketosis, called the keto flu, as your body adapts to the new diet, but not everyone experiences it the same way.

WHAT IS THE KETO FLU?

As your body makes its transition from burning carbs to burning fat, it takes a few days to adapt. This can vary anywhere between 3 to 15 days depending on your body, metabolism, and insulin sensitivity. In these early days, it's not uncommon to feel a sense of malaise and some fatigue, and occasionally headaches. This is also because of loss of electrolytes, because the keto diet can be diuretic. Carbs hold on to water, and as you reduce your carb intake, your body's water retention also reduces. But don't let the keto flu scare you: it fades within a couple of days. The best way to combat it is by drinking electrolyte-rich drinks like soup or chicken stock; even a bouillon cube in water will work in a pinch. Most people, though, won't experience the flu at all, and will be able to transition into ketosis effortlessly.

CAN I HAVE A CHEAT DAY ON KETO?

Unlike other diets, keto is an all or nothing process. Eat too many carbs and you'll kick yourself right out of ketosis, and you'll have to begin the process of getting into it all over again. As a rule, it's best not to cheat at all, at least in the first month of the diet.

But as your body becomes more keto adapted, you'll find it's easier to slip into ketosis, at which point the occasional cheat day won't hurt. They've also been known to break a weight stall after a few months of keto adaptation.

And though the idea of a cheat day may sound great, you'll often find that going back to processed carbs and sugar actually makes you more miserable than happy. You want to cheat responsibly, to not turn a cheat meal into a cheat day, and a cheat day into a cheat week. Cheat rarely, and cheat well, perhaps throwing in complex carbs and whole grain food into your day, instead of diving head first into a bag of chips or a tub of ice cream.

IS ALCOHOL ALLOWED ON THE KETO DIET?

Ideally, alcohol is best avoided, as it can hamper weight loss irrespective of the diet you are on. However, occasionally you may find yourself in a social situation where you can't (or don't want to) turn down a drink. Are there keto-safe drinks? Yes. Most distilled spirits, like whiskey, white rum, cognac, vodka, and tequila are virtually carb-free. You want to be careful with dark rum, because it can contain a significant amount of sugar. Sweet liqueurs and beers are total no-nos (even the light beers have enough carbs to swallow up your entire day's allowance), as are sugared sodas. If you must drink chasers, pick sugar-free sodas and mixers. And while you can indulge in a glass or two of dry red or white wine, it's best not to exceed that amount, given that, on average, a glass of wine would contain close to 3 grams of carbs.

It's also important to note that on keto, the alcohol is likely to hit you much quicker and harder and hangovers can be significantly worse, because you don't have carbs to buffer it with, so it's essential to drink plenty of water with your alcohol. The most important thing to remember, though, is that alcohol is adding no nutrition, only empty calories to your diet, so weigh

THE KETO DOS AND DON'TS

DON'T THINK OF KETO AS A MAGIC DIET

While the keto diet does turn your body into a fat burning machine, it's important to not think that will magic away fat overnight. Yes, the keto diet works faster and more visibly than some other diets, and you may lose more initial weight with it, but it's important to exercise control and stick to your macros to see results. The initial, very quick, weight drop is often just water weight, so it's normal to find your weight stalling and weight loss slowing a bit after the first few pounds. It's also important to realize that everybody is unique and the diet will work differently for different people.

DON'T OBSESS OVER THE SCALE

Often, people get too caught up with the weighing scale. Keto is so much more than a number on a scale; it impacts how you feel and your overall well being. Sometimes people lose inches rather than weight while on keto; often, your body is losing fat and gaining muscle. There are various reasons the numbers on the scale may not drop, but if you are feeling good, losing inches, and overall getting the benefits of being on keto, it's best to keep the scale obsession to a minimum.

DO EAT LOTS OF REAL FOOD

It's important on the keto diet (and life in general) to eat good quality food. Fresh vegetables, meat, and dairy are so much healthier than their packaged and processed counterparts. If you eat good food, you will feel good.

DO COUNT YOUR MACROS

Being committed and having discipline definitely yields better results. It's very important to know how much you are eating and whether you are getting in the right amount of fats, protein, and carbs from the food you eat. If you aren't hitting your macros enough, there's a chance you'll be left hungry and craving unhealthy food. Monitoring your macros makes for more steady and disciplined weight loss.

DRINK LOTS OF WATER

This cannot be stressed enough. It's extremely important to stay hydrated and drink plenty of water while you are on the keto diet. Since your body is not holding on to any water, you need to keep your reserves replenished. Drink at least two litres a day, if not more. And if you don't fancy plain water, it's amazing what a slice of lime or a few cucumber slices can do to the taste.

DON'T OVEREAT

While there is a lot of debate about whether calories matter on this diet, it's important to realize that if you stuff your face and overeat, no matter what diet you do, it won't work. If you are eating more food than your body requires, you're not helping it shed weight.

DON'T EAT PROCESSED/ PACKAGED FOOD

Most processed food isn't good for you. There's significant deterioration in the quality of macronutrients when food is over processed and packaged food always has a lot of insidious hidden carbs. It's best to eat as much fresh produce as possible and cook most, if not all, of your own food. Also processed/packaged foods like peanut butter and mayonnaise, which are keto friendly, are still best made on your own as most supermarket brands will have sugar included or ingredients like palm oil that you want to avoid.

DO CHECK THE NUTRITIONAL INFO OF ALL FOOD YOU EAT

Always check the nutritional labels on items before you eat them. Lots of brands are often misleading with their advertising so it's important to check the nutritional label for carb content as well as for the ingredients that are there. Even with fresh produce like vegetables, if you find yourself in doubt, a quick search on the internet can help you find the nutritional information for the item. It's always better to be safe than sorry.

DO USE NATURAL SUGAR FREE OPTIONS

When it comes to sugar-free sweetener options, it can get pretty confusing because there are currently a lot of different variants in the market. Some of these are keto safe, like erythritol and Stevia. Most others are best avoided, as they either have high glycemic indexes that can cause your insulin to spike, or are just generally deemed unhealthy. Sugar alcohols like maltitol and xylitol have high GIs and are not advised. Natural sugars like coconut sugar and agave nectar and even honey trigger insulin just like white sugar, so they're completely off the table on this diet. Once in a while, it's not a big deal if you drink a diet soda with aspartame, it's best to try and stick to more natural sugar substitutes like Stevia.

DON'T GO OVERBOARD ON THE FAT

For some reason, when people think high fat, they assume it's eating sticks of butter. This couldn't be further from the truth. It's important to incorporate good fat sources into your diet but, when it comes to weight loss, it's also important to have an overall calorie deficit, so your body can burn its own fat for fuel. So, for weight loss, it's important to maintain this deficit and encourage your body to burn its own fat.

KETOGENICS 101

BREAKFAST

Nothing gets you up and out of bed like the thought of a good breakfast. On keto, you can really indulge yourself for breakfast – think eggs and ham, cheese, bacon. Eggs, you will discover, are your keto best friends, packed full of good fats and highly nutritious... and it helps that they're so wildly versatile. Other than all the poaching, scrambling, frying they lend themselves to, they're also great vehicles for leftovers – you can make a frittata of most things lying in your refrigerator, be it leftover roast chicken, sautéed vegetables or even meatloaf scraps. It's the blank canvas for you to paint your culinary skills on.

On the ketogenic diet, breakfast goes a long way towards getting a good portion of your fats and proteins in. Not only does it add significantly to your daily macros, it also keeps you satiated, so hunger pangs don't kick in and have you reaching for that rogue mid-morning cookie. These recipes are easily customizable, so feel free to add in whatever you fancy (whatever fits in the ketogenic diet, that is). And with so many to choose from, you're going to be spoilt for choice. Don't skip breakfast; it's the fastest way to a happy keto day.

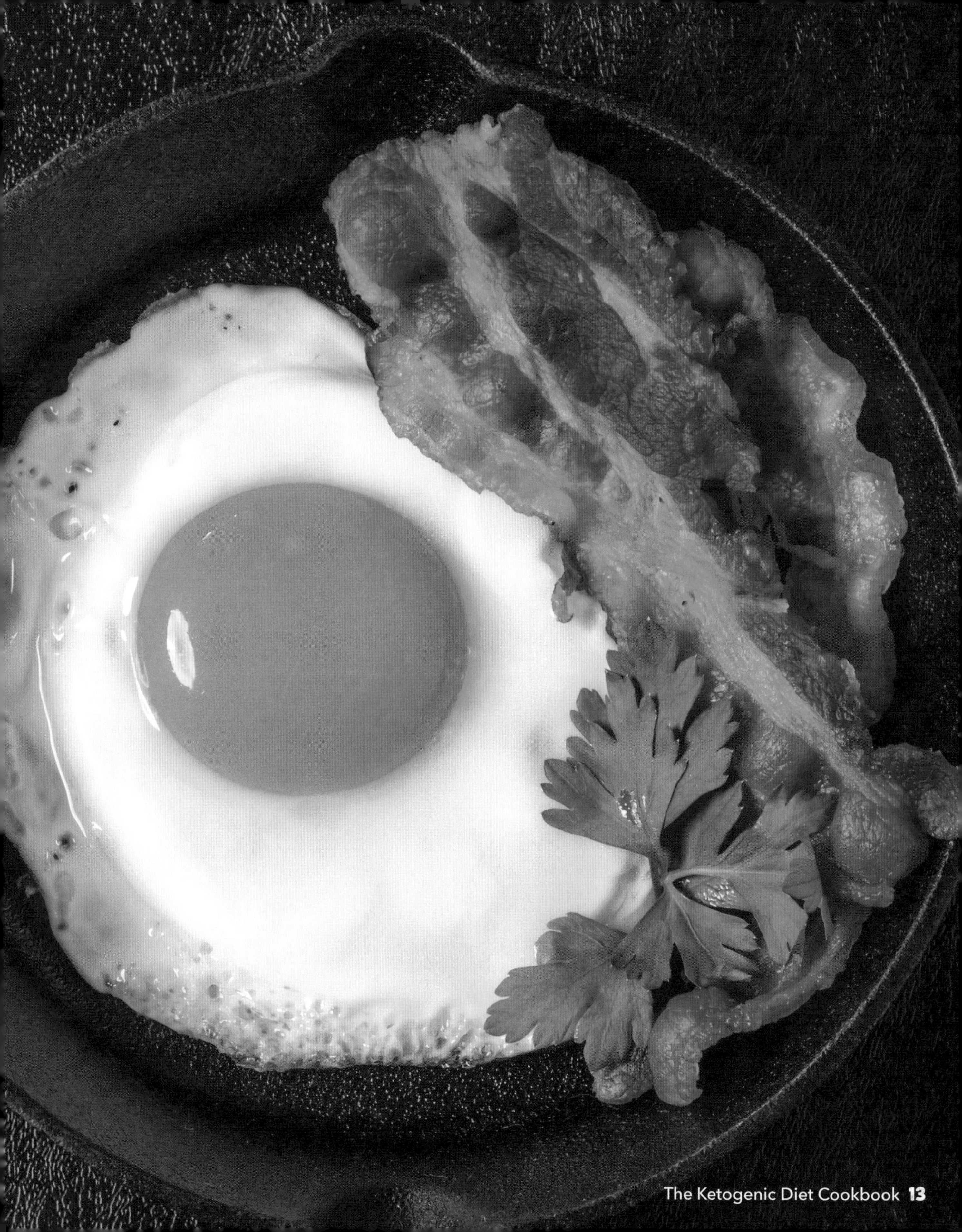

CHEESY SCRAMBLED EGGS

SERVES: 2 / CALORIES: 728 / FAT: 63G / NET CARBS: 3G / PROTEIN: 38G

2 tablespoons butter

6 large eggs

¼ cup heavy cream

1 cup shredded sharp cheddar cheese

½ teaspoon salt

Freshly ground black pepper

1. Heat the skillet over medium-high heat. Melt the butter in the skillet, being careful not to let it burn.

2. In a bowl, whisk the eggs until combined. Add the cream and whisk it into the eggs. Pour the egg mixture into the hot skillet. Using a wooden spoon, start to stir the eggs in the skillet as they start to cook. After a couple of minutes, turn the heat down to medium. Top the eggs with the cheese and stir it in as the eggs finish cooking. Be careful not to overcook the eggs.

3. Remove from heat, add salt and pepper, and serve immediately. Season with additional salt and pepper to taste.

BIG TIP

This is gooey goodness at its best. Well, you could always add bacon crumbles to take it way over the top, but the egg-and-cheese combo is pretty darn perfect in its simplicity.

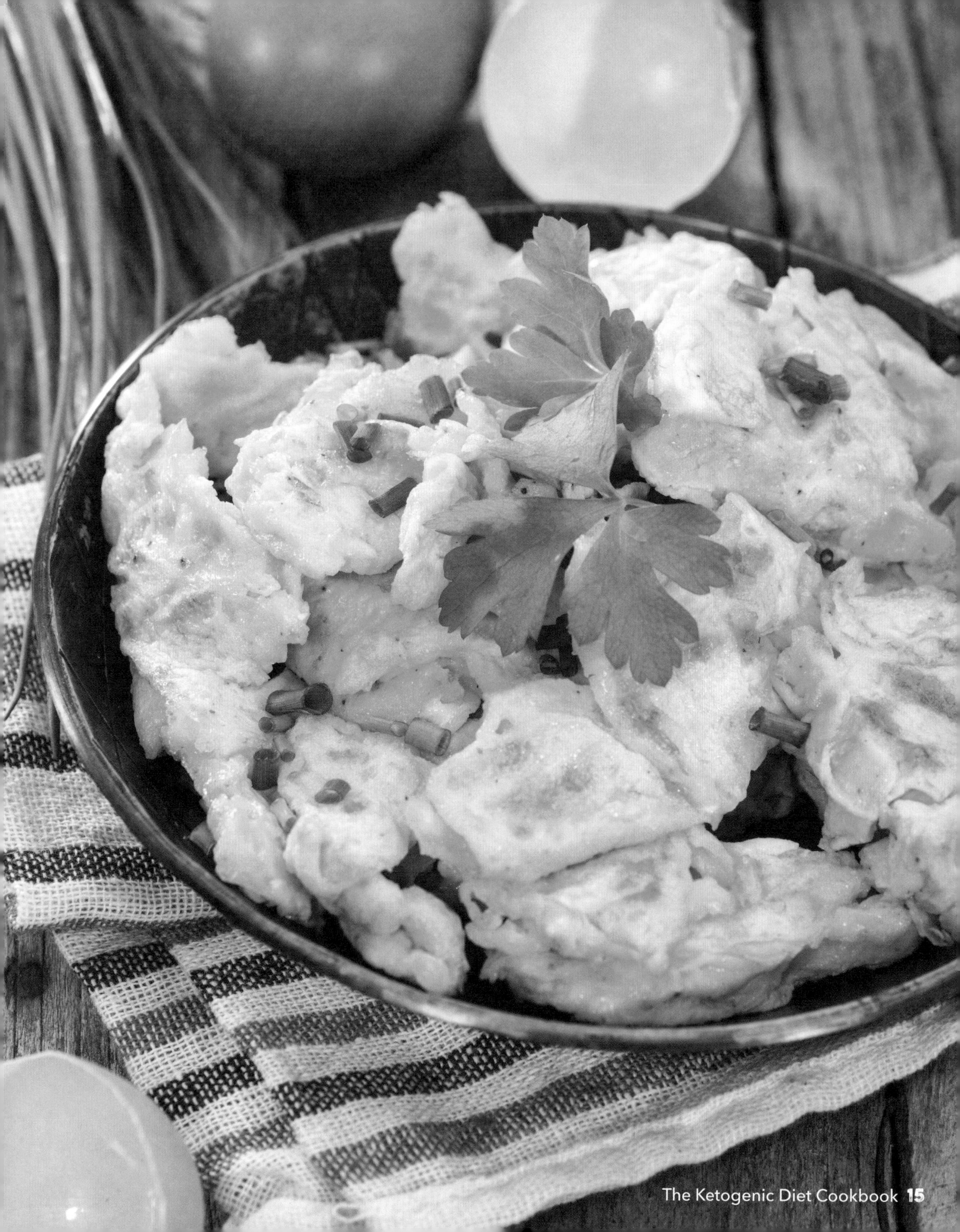

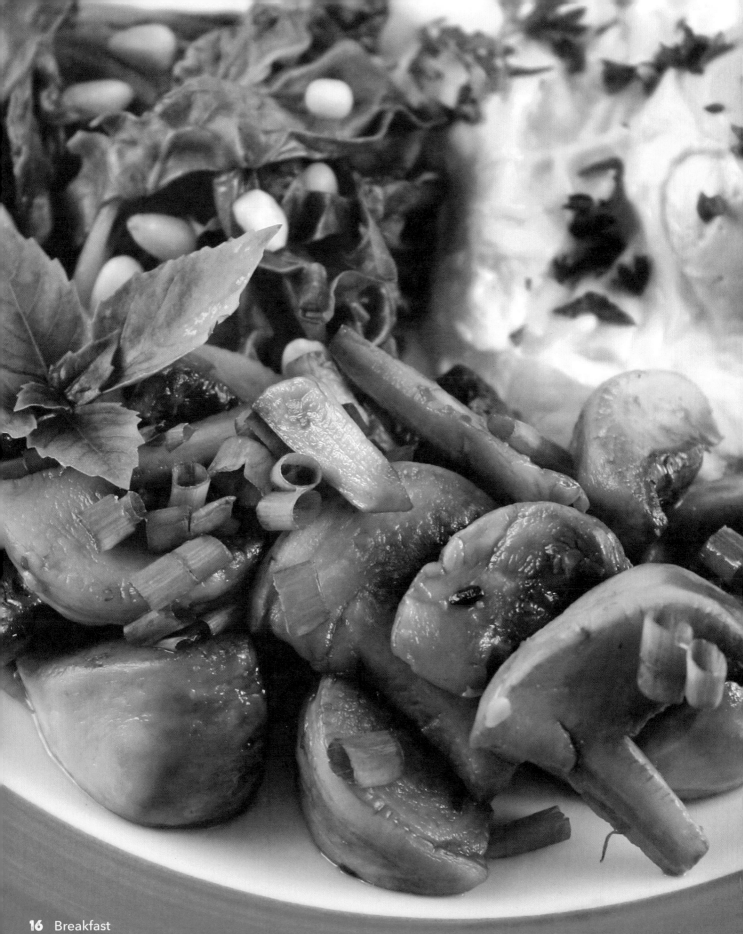

EGG BAKE WITH SPINACH AND MUSHROOM

SERVES: 6 / CALORIES: 371 / FAT: 30G / NET CARBS: 5G / PROTEIN: 18G

2 tablespoons extra virgin olive oil

1 cup onion, chopped fine

1 cup sliced domestic mushrooms

4 cups spinach leaves, coarse stems removed, and ripped or cut into smaller pieces

12 eggs

1 cup heavy cream

1 tablespoon chopped fresh parsley

Salt and pepper to taste

1. Lightly grease the inside of the slow cooker with a teaspoon of the extra virgin olive oil. In large skillet, cook onion and mushrooms in remainder of olive oil until tender. Turn the heat off, place the spinach leaves over the mixture, and cover with a tight-fitting lid. Allow the spinach to steam under the lid for about 10 minutes, which will cause it to wilt.

2. In a large bowl, beat the eggs with the heavy cream until well mixed. Add the onion, mushroom, and spinach mixture, then the parsley, and stir just to combine.

3. Pour the eggs and vegetables into the slow cooker, cover and turn on low. Cook for 1 to 2 hours, until eggs are thoroughly cooked. To test for doneness, insert a clean knife in the center. If it comes out clean, the dish is ready.

BIG TIP

This is delicious served with a fresh salsa. Chop 2 very ripe tomatoes and put them in a small bowl. Add a squirt of lime juice, a tablespoon of finely minced onion, 1 clove of crushed garlic, and a teaspoon or so of chopped jalapeno pepper (or a spicy pepper of your choice). Season with pepper and just a dash of salt.

BROCCOLI FRITTATA

SERVES: 4 / CALORIES: 282 / FAT: 22G / NET CARBS: 4G / PROTEIN: 15G

2 tablespoons extra virgin olive oil

4 tablespoons onion, chopped

2 cloves garlic, minced

½ red or green bell pepper,
seeds and ribs removed, thinly sliced

8 large eggs

4 tablespoons heavy cream

2 tablespoons fresh chopped parsley

1 tablespoon fresh thyme

¾ cup fresh broccoli florets, cut into
bite-sized pieces

1. Heat the extra virgin olive oil in a skillet and add onion, garlic, and bell pepper. Cook over medium-high heat until onion is translucent, about 3 minutes.

2. In a large bowl, whisk eggs with heavy cream, then add herbs and broccoli pieces. Add the cooked vegetables. Take a large piece of parchment paper, fold it in half, and place it in the slow cooker so the sides come up the sides of the cooker. This will give you a way to lift out the egg dish when it is cooked. Pour the egg mixture in on top of the parchment paper.

3. Cover and cook on High for about 1 hour or on Low for closer to 2 hours until eggs are set.

4. Run a spatula along the sides of the cooker to loosen the parchment paper. Lift the frittata out of the cooker with the paper, and slide it onto a serving plate.

BIG TIP

Broccoli is loaded with Vitamin C and dietary fiber.

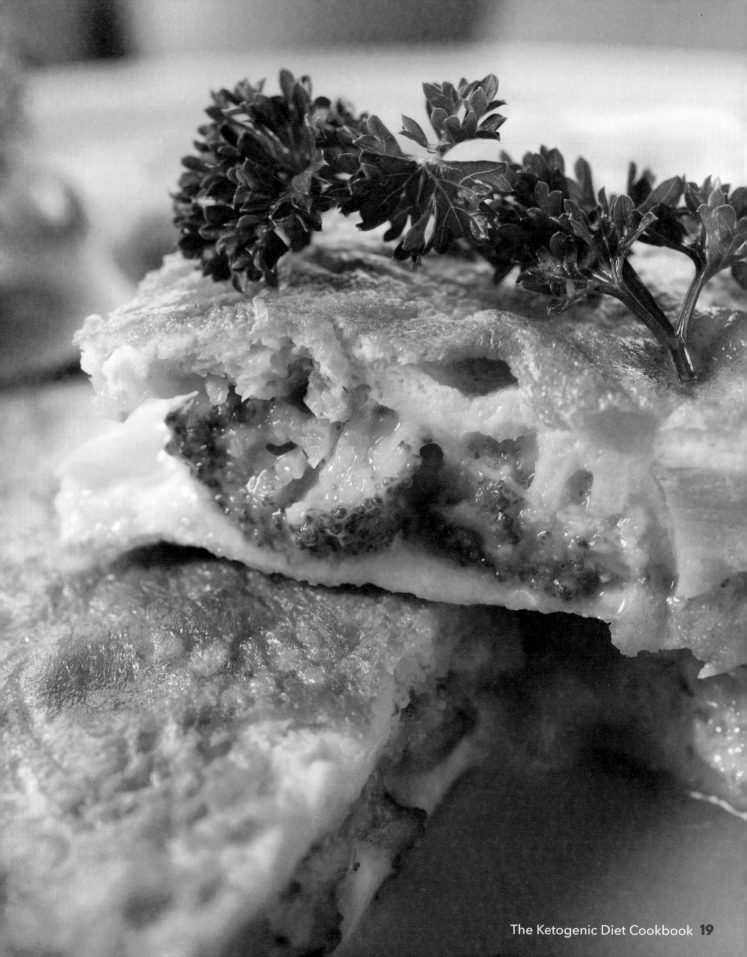

CORNED BEEF HASH AND EGGS

SERVES: 4 / CALORIES: 351 / FAT: 27G / NET CARBS: 4G / PROTEIN: 21G

3 tablespoons butter

¼ cup onion, chopped fine

1 clove garlic, minced

2 cups cauliflower florets, diced

1 pound corned beef, shredded

¼ cup chicken broth

2 eggs

Salt and pepper to taste

Non-stick cooking spray

1. In a skillet over medium-high heat, melt the butter. Add the onion and garlic and cook, stirring, until the onion is wilted, about 1 minute. Stir in the cauliflower pieces and stir, warming them through. Remove the pan from the heat.

2. Coat the inside of the slow cooker with non-stick cooking spray, and put the cauliflower mixture inside. Stir in the corned beef. Pour the chicken broth over everything. Cover and cook on Low for 1 hour 20 minutes, on High for about 45 to 60 minutes. Season with salt and pepper to taste. Serve hot.

BIG TIP

Corned Beef Hash and Eggs: For an even more filling breakfast, add eggs. Simply crack two eggs open over the hash mixture in the slow cooker before cooking. They will cook along with the hash. Factor in an additional 20 to 30 minutes on Low or 15 to 30 on High.

MAINLY MUSHROOM FRITATA

SERVES: 4 / CALORIES: 486 / FAT: 39G / NET CARBS: 8G / PROTEIN: 26G

3 tablespoons butter

½ cup onion, diced

1 pound mushrooms, picked over and sliced or chopped

1 teaspoon salt

½ teaspoon pepper

8 eggs

½ cup heavy cream

1 cup Swiss cheese, shredded

⅓ cup fresh parsley, chopped

1. Melt the butter in the skillet over medium-high heat. Add the onions and cook, stirring, until translucent, about 3 minutes. Add the mushrooms, lower the heat slightly, and cook, stirring occasionally, until soft, 5 to 10 minutes. Drain the liquid from the pan. Season the mushrooms with the salt and pepper.

2. In a bowl, whisk the eggs with the milk. Pour the egg mixture over the mushrooms. Sprinkle the cheese all around the top, and then sprinkle the parsley over everything. Cover the skillet and let cook until set, about 10 minutes. Place the skillet in the oven under the broiler and "toast" the top, about 2 minutes.

BIG TIP

The selection of mushrooms in grocery stores is getting bigger and bigger. You can use one kind of mushroom for this dish, or you can use several kinds together.

EARLY RISER POACHED SALMON

SERVES: 4 / CALORIES: 643 / FAT: 44G / NET CARBS: 5G / PROTEIN: 51G

6 cups water

½ cup onion, chopped

½ cup celery, chopped

4 sprigs parsley

½ cup freshly squeezed lemon juice

8 whole black peppercorns

1 bay leaf

4 small steaks of salmon (8oz each filet)

4 tablespoons salted butter

1 small lemon, sliced, for garnish

2 tablespoons fresh parsley, chopped, for garnish

1. To prep the poaching liquid, combine water, onion, celery, parsley, lemon juice, peppercorns, and bay leaf over medium heat. Bring to a boil and simmer for 30 minutes. Strain and discard solids.

2. Take a large sheet of heavy duty aluminum foil and place it inside the slow cooker so the sides emerge over the top. Press it into place so it conforms with the inside of the cooker. Turn the cooker on to High and, uncovered, let it preheat. Place the salmon over the foil in the slow cooker. Pour the hot poaching liquid over the salmon. Cover immediately, and cook on High for 1 to 2 hours until the flesh of the salmon is cooked through to a light pink but firm color and consistency.

3. Remove stoneware from slow cooker. Allow salmon to cool for 20 minutes before transferring to a platter and serving.

4. Melt the butter and pour a tablespoon over each filet before serving.

5. Garnish with lemon slices and fresh parsley sprigs.

BIG TIP

This is a really tasty and satisfying breakfast after a workout, especially an early morning run. Imagine coming home to a fragrant, succulent piece of hot salmon. Mmm.

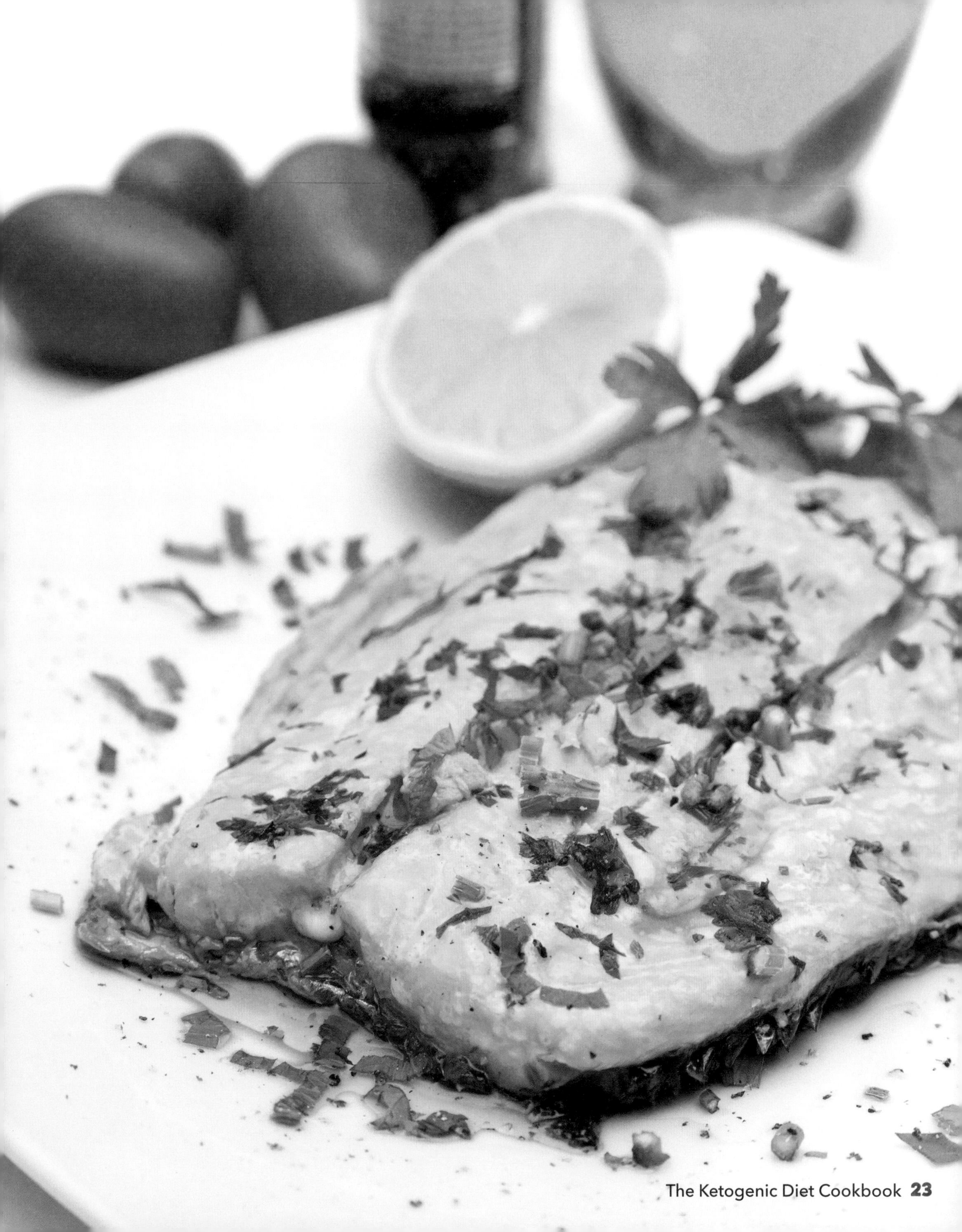

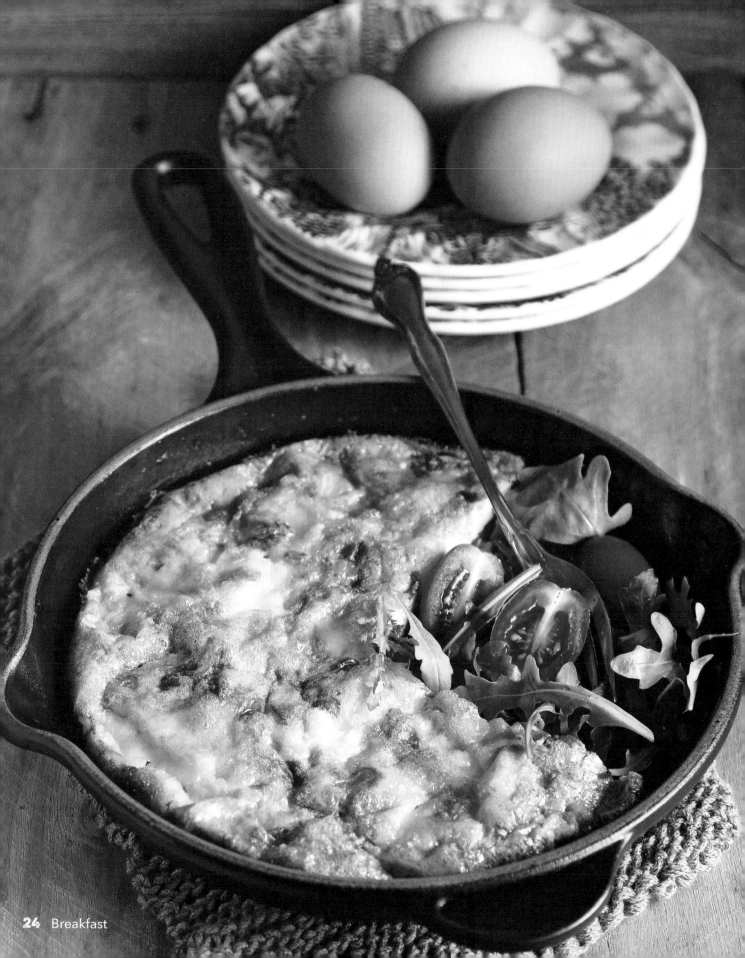

SPINACH FRITTATA

SERVES: 4 / CALORIES: 237 / FAT: 18G / NET CARBS: 3G / PROTEIN: 15G

6 eggs

2 tablespoons butter

¼ cup chopped red onion

1 clove garlic, minced

2 cups fresh spinach leaves, coarse stems removed, roughly chopped

½ cup feta cheese

Salt and pepper to taste

1. Preheat the broiler to low.

2. In a small bowl, beat the eggs with a whisk until combined.

3. Heat skillet over medium-high heat. Melt the butter in the skillet and add the onions and garlic, stirring to cook until onions are translucent, about 3 minutes.

4. Add the spinach and stir so the leaves wilt. Sprinkle the feta over the mixture.

5. Pour the eggs over everything and shake the pan to evenly distribute them. Sprinkle with salt and pepper. Cover the skillet and let cook until set, about 10 minutes. Place the skillet in the oven under the broiler to "toast" the top, about 2 minutes.

6. Allow to stand for a couple of minutes, and serve. Season with additional salt and pepper to taste.

GARDEN VEGETABLE EGGS

SERVES: 4 / CALORIES: 326 / FAT: 28G / NET CARBS: 5G / PROTEIN: 14G

2 tablespoons olive oil

4oz onion, chopped fine

4oz small zucchini, chopped

4oz small green pepper, deseeded and chopped

4oz ripe plum tomatoes, chopped

¼ cup chopped fresh basil

8 eggs

½ cup heavy cream

Salt and pepper to taste

1. Lightly grease the inside of the slow cooker with a teaspoon of the olive oil. In large skillet, cook onion, zucchini, and pepper until just tender, about 5 minutes. Add the tomatoes and basil and stir to heat through. Remove from heat.

2. In a large bowl, beat the eggs and heavy cream until well mixed. Add the vegetable mixture, and stir just to combine. Pour the eggs and vegetables into the slow cooker, cover and turn on low. Cook for 1 to 2 hours, until eggs are thoroughly cooked. To test for doneness, insert a clean knife in the center. If it comes out clean, the dish is ready.

BIG TIP

Eggs Benedict: Create a gourmet low-carb version of eggs Benedict by serving this yummy egg dish on top of a slice of keto toasted bread, with a piece of grilled Canadian bacon and a dollop of homemade hollandaise sauce. When the egg dish has about a half hour left, make the hollandaise by whisking 3 egg yolks with 1 tablespoon each water and lemon juice in a small saucepan until well combined. Put the saucepan over low heat and keep mixing, cooking for about 5 minutes until mixture gets frothy and light. Remove the pan from the heat and stir in 6 tablespoons of butter, one at a time. Season with salt and pepper and a dash of cayenne.

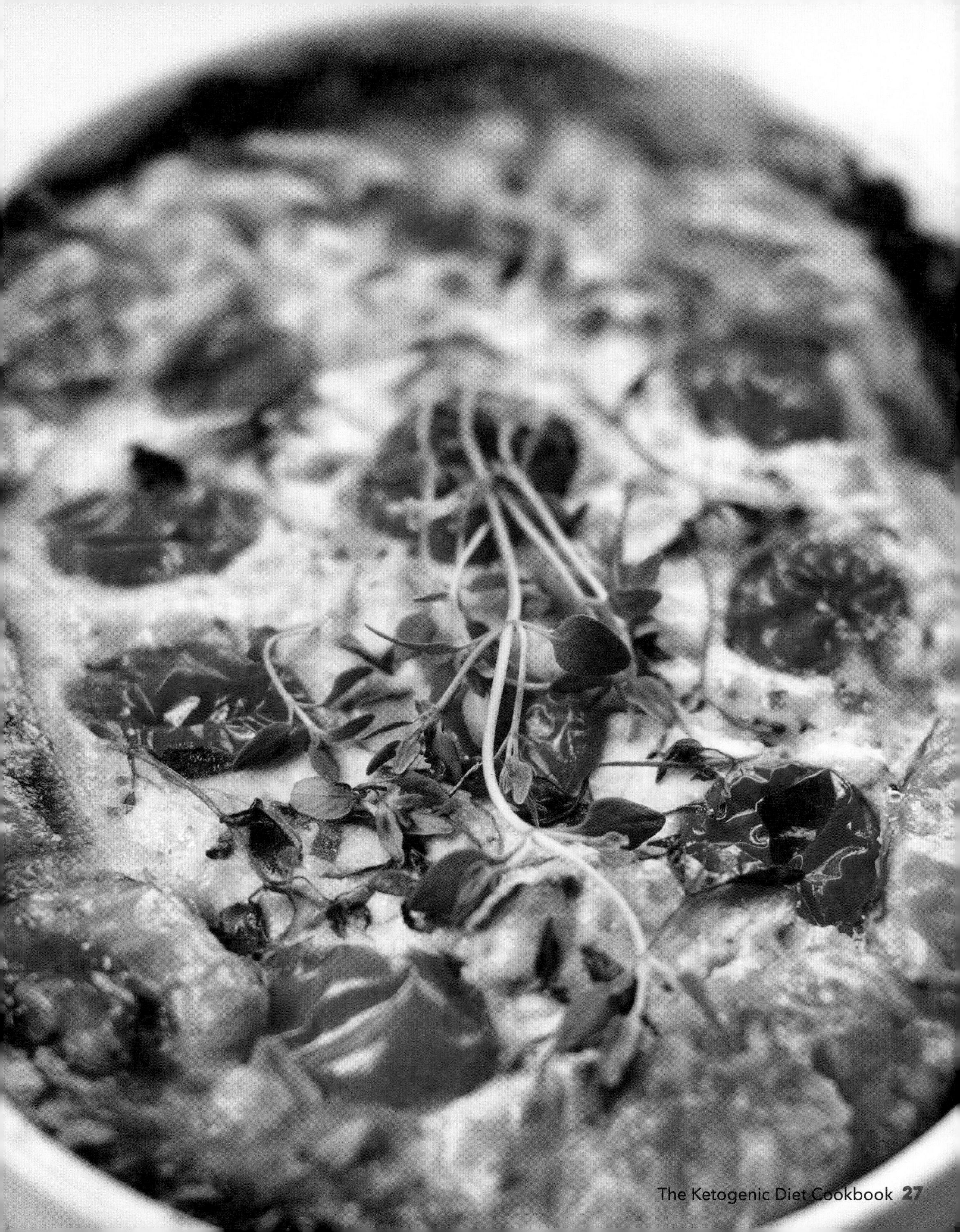

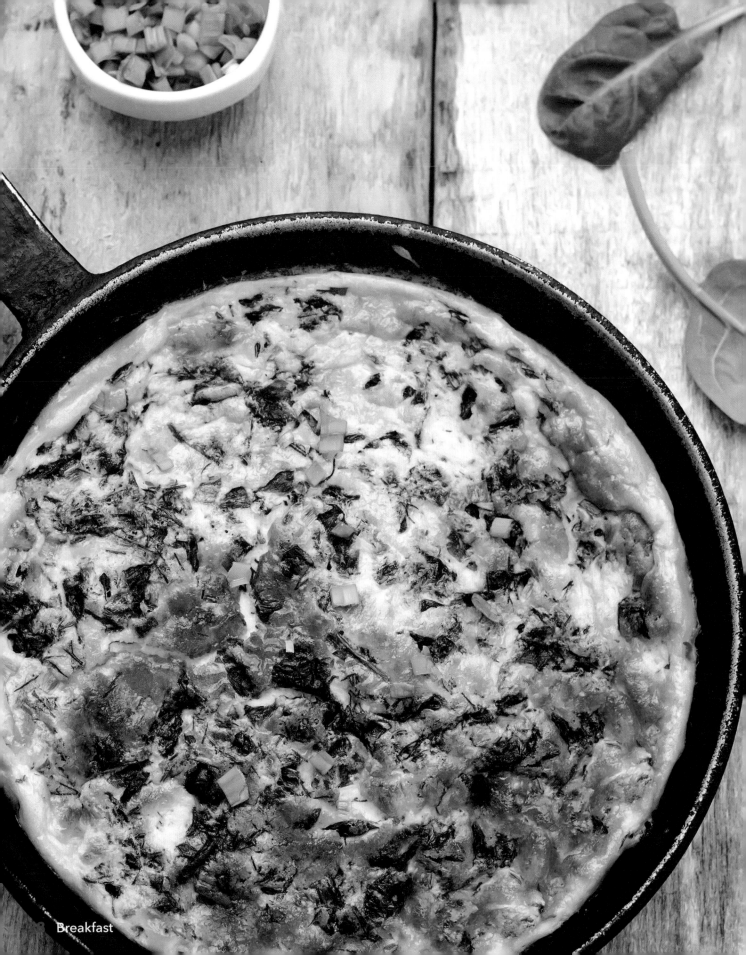

Breakfast

GREEN EGGS AND HAM

SERVES: 2 / CALORIES: 573 / FAT: 48G / NET CARBS: 6G / PROTEIN: 30G

1 tablespoon olive oil

3.5oz cooked ham, cut into pieces

6 eggs

½ cup heavy cream

½ cup steamed spinach, chopped, excess water squeezed out

2 tablespoons fresh parsley, chopped

Salt and pepper to taste

1. In a small skillet, heat the olive oil over medium-high heat. Add the ham to coat with the oil and brown slightly, about a minute. Remove from heat.

2. In a large bowl, beat the eggs with the heavy cream until well blended. Add the spinach and parsley, and whisk to combine everything well and break up the spinach pieces.

3. Place the ham in the slow cooker, and pour the eggs over top. Cover and cook on Low for about 1 hour, until the eggs are cooked through. Season with salt and pepper when serving.

BIG TIP

The Dr. Seuss book *Green Eggs and Ham* was produced as a result of a bet between the prolific author/illustrator and his equally accomplished editor, Bennett Cerf. Cerf's challenge was that Seuss use no more than 50 words in the entire book.

CRUSTLESS QUICHE

SERVES: 6 / CALORIES: 411 / FAT: 36G / NET CARBS: 4G / 17G PROTEIN

4 tablespoons unsalted butter

½ cup onion, sliced into ribbons

2 cups sliced fresh mushrooms
(this can be any kind of mushrooms from
domestic to Portobello, crimini, shiitake,
or any combination)

½ teaspoon dried sage

Salt and pepper to taste

10 eggs, beaten

1 cup heavy cream

1 cup shredded Swiss cheese

1. In a skillet over medium-high heat, melt the butter. Add the onions and stir until wilted, about 2 minutes. Add the mushroom slices and stir, cooking, until they start to soften and shrink, about 5 minutes. Remove from heat. Drain any liquid produced by the mushrooms. Stir in the sage, and season with salt and pepper.

2. In a bowl, beat the eggs. Add the heavy cream and the cheese, and then add the mushroom and onion mix.

3. Transfer everything to the slow cooker. Cover and cook on Low for 4 hours, being careful not to overcook. Serve hot.

BIG TIP

If you want to add meat to this recipe, sauté some turkey bacon
until crumbly. Add it to the mushroom mixture before cooking,
or sprinkle it on top at the end.

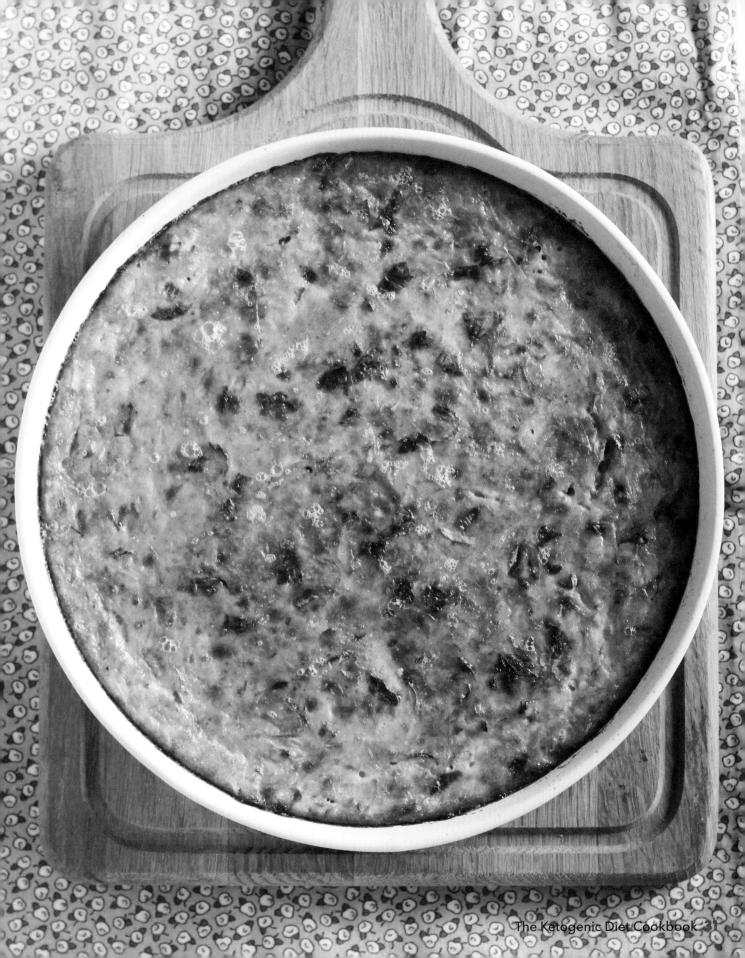

SOUPS & STEWS

If you're on the ketogenic diet, you'll find you're doing a lot more cooking if you want to avoid the hidden carbs in store-bought food and even restaurant meals. This is where soups and stews step in. For starters, they're great comfort food – there's nothing quite like wolfing down a bowl of hot soup on a cold winter day. More importantly, they're effortless to make, don't take up too many pots and pans, and are still complete one-bowl meals.

For soups and stews, it's good to know how to make a great stock, because that forms the base of both. It's also a great way to get your vegetables in, something we tend to miss out on on keto because we're trying to up our fat and protein macros. Veggies are important because they give you nutrients and vitamins that you're not going to get just from meat and dairy. They're also your main source of carbohydrates on this diet, just enough to balance out your macros.

As for stews, they're some of most flavorful dishes that can be created using the cheaper and tougher cuts of meat. The slow cooking process allows the meat to break down and the flavor to really build up. Okay, so you can't mop it all up with bread, but some keto bread or cauliflower rice makes for a perfect accompaniment. And these are so tasty, you can just eat them as is.

Throw a stew or soup on, let it simmer and fill your home with its lovely aromas, while you go about doing your chores. Who said keto is hard?

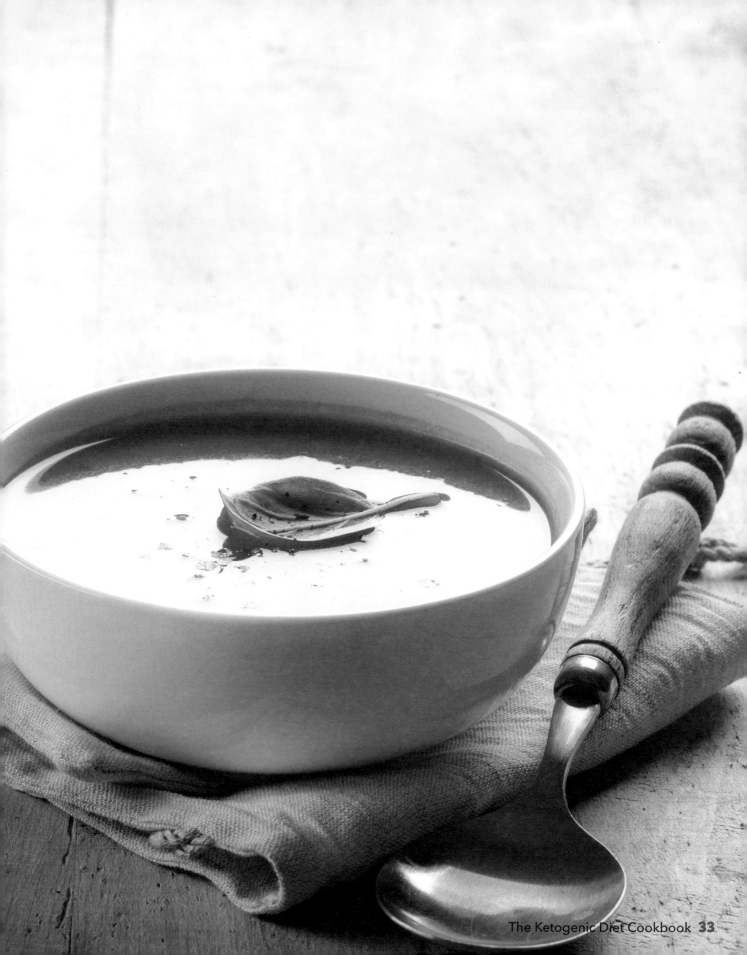

BEEF STOCK

MAKES 10 CUPS / CALORIES: 31 / FAT: 2G / NET CARBS: 0G / PROTEIN: 5G

2 lbs beef marrow bones

2 lbs meaty rib or neck bones

3 quarts water

¼ cup vinegar

3 sprigs of fresh thyme

1 teaspoon peppercorns

1 bunch parsley

1. Place the beef bones in a large pot and cover with water and vinegar. Let stand for one hour.

2. Place the meaty bones in a roasting pan. Preheat the oven to 350 and roast until well browned, about 30 to 40 minutes.

3. Place the soaked beef bones and the browned pieces in the slow cooker. Add the thyme and peppercorns, and cover with the water.

4. Discard the fat from the roasting pan, and fill with an inch or so of water. Place the pan over a burner on medium-high heat, and as the water heats, stir to loosen the coagulated juices and browned bits. Add this to the slow cooker. The water should just cover the meat; add more if it doesn't.

5. Turn the slow cooker on High and cook for 2 to 3 hours until liquid is boiling. Remove lid and scoop out and discard scum that has risen to the top.

6. Replace the lid, lower the heat to Low, and cook for 12 to 18 hours–the longer, the better. Add the parsley during the last 15 minutes.

7. When cooking is complete, remove the solids with a slotted spoon into a colander over a bowl. Any drippings in the bowl can go back into the stock. Remove any meat from the bones and eat separately.

8. Transfer the stock to a large bowl and refrigerate. When the fat is congealed on top, remove it, and transfer the stock to several smaller containers with tight-fitting lids. Stock can be stored in the refrigerator for several days, or kept frozen.

BIG TIP

Before you begin, be aware that stocks cook slower– that is, all day. Ideally, leave the fat in the stock since it's good fat that we need, or use it for cooking.

FISH STOCK

MAKES 10 CUPS / CALORIES: 41 / FAT: 2G / NET CARBS: 0G / PROTEIN: 5G

2 tablespoons clarified butter

3 quarts cold water

¼ cup vinegar

3 sprigs fresh thyme

Several sprigs fresh parsley

1 bay leaf

2 or 3 whole carcasses from non-oily fish such as snapper, rockfish, sole, or cod

1. Place the carcasses in the slow cooker. Cover with the water and vinegar. Add the bay leaf.

2. Cover and cook on High for 4 to 5 hours until liquid is boiling. Remove the cover and scoop off and discard the scum that has risen to the top.

3. Replace the cover and cook on Low for 10 to 18 hours—the longer the better.

4. When cooking is complete, remove the solids with a slotted spoon. Transfer the stock to a large bowl and refrigerate. When the fat is congealed on top, remove it, and transfer the stock to several smaller containers with tight-fitting lids. Stock can be stored in the refrigerator for several days, or kept frozen.

BIG TIP

Make a more delicate seafood stock using lobster bodies from which the claws and tail have been removed. For this recipe, use 3 to 4 lobster bodies, or the bodies of 2 lobsters and the shells from 2 to 4 pounds of raw shrimp.

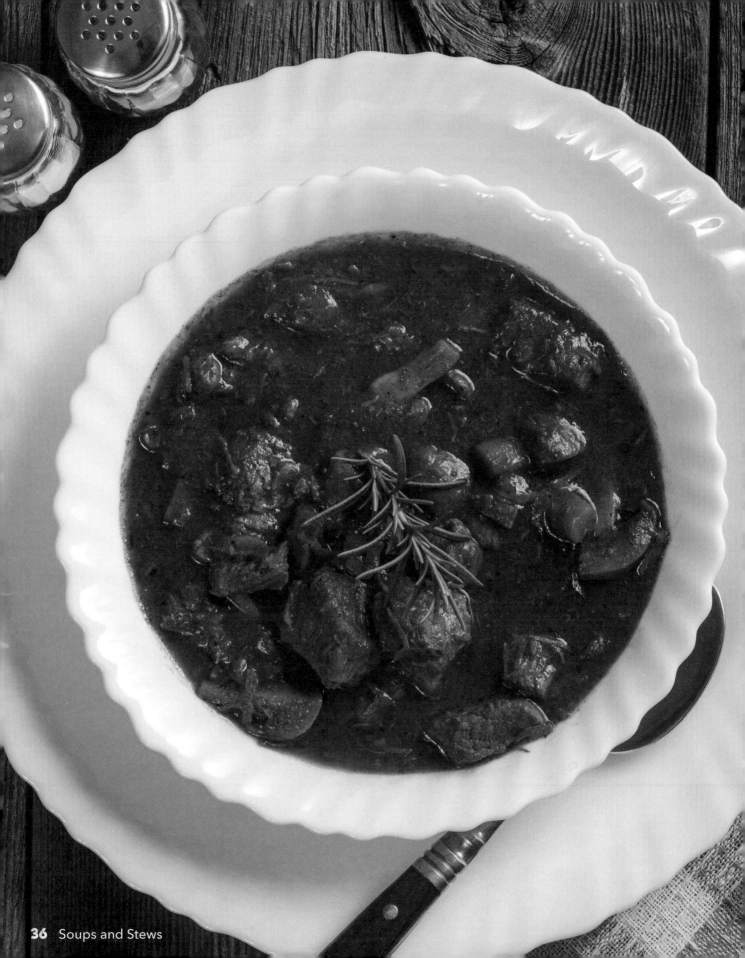

WINE- NOT BEEF STEW

SERVES: 8 / CALORIES: 398 / FAT: 17G / NET CARBS: 12G / PROTEIN: 50G

4 tablespoons olive oil

2 cloves garlic, minced

4 lbs beef stew meat

1 onion, sliced thin

½ cup fresh mushrooms, sliced

1 teaspoon dried rosemary

Salt and pepper to taste

1 cup dry red wine

2 cups water

1. Heat the oil in a skillet and add the garlic. Brown the stew pieces in the oil until lightly browned on all sides. Transfer to the slow cooker.

2. Add the onion to the skillet and cook, stirring, until onions are translucent, about 3 minutes. Add the mushrooms and stir, cooking, another minute or so. Remove from heat and add the rosemary. Season the mushroom/onion mix with salt and freshly ground pepper. Add to the slow cooker.

3. Pour the wine and water over everything in the slow cooker. Cover and cook on Low for 8 to 10 hours or on High for 6 to 7 hours.

BIG TIP

Since this dish has more protein than fat, it would make sense to add a tablespoon of butter per portion to add more fat if required to hit your daily macros. At 12 net carbs, this dish is a bit higher than most keto dishes but if you make the stew without the wine, it will result in a much lower carb stew.

CHICKEN SOUP WITH FENNEL

SERVES: 8 / CALORIES: 162 / FAT: 10G / NET CARBS: 5G / PROTEIN: 14G

1 lb boneless, skinless chicken thighs

1 large fennel bulb

4 tablespoons extra virgin olive oil

4 oz onions, diced

3 garlic cloves, minced

5 cups chicken stock or broth

14 oz tomatoes, pureed in the food processor

2 teaspoon fennel seeds, crushed

Salt and pepper to taste

1. Rinse the chicken and pat dry with paper towels. Cut into ½-inch cubes. Rinse the fennel and cut in half lengthwise. Discard core and ribs, and dice bulb into ¾-inch pieces. Place the chicken and fennel in the slow cooker.

2. Heat olive oil in a medium skillet over medium-high heat. Add onions and garlic and cook, stirring frequently, until onions are translucent, about 3 minutes. Scrape mixture into slow cooker.

3. Stir stock, tomatoes (with juice), and fennel seeds into the slow cooker and stir to combine all ingredients. Cover and cook on Low for 5 to 7 hours or on High for 2½ to 3 hours, or until chicken is cooked through and tender.

4. If cooking on Low, raise the heat to High. Season to taste with salt and pepper, and serve hot.

BIG TIP

Fresh fennel, finocchio in Italian, and sometimes called anise in supermarkets, has a slightly licorice taste but the texture of celery, both raw and cooked. You can always substitute 2 celery ribs for each ½ fennel bulb specified in a recipe. This recipe has a lower fat content and can be finished with a tablespoon of olive oil or butter to help you hit your fat macros if needed.

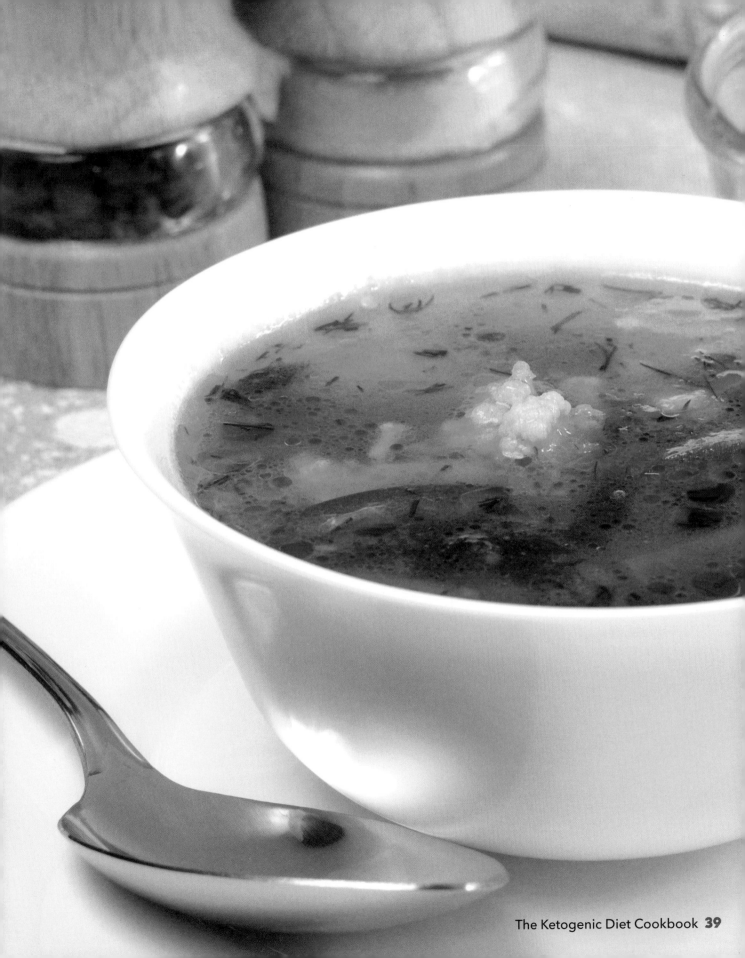

PORTUGUESE KALE AND SAUSAGE SOUP

SERVES: 6 / CALORIES: 281 / FAT: 21G / NET CARBS: 8G / PROTEIN: 18G

2 tablespoons olive oil

4 oz onion, finely chopped

1 garlic clove, finely chopped

¾ pound homemade pork sausage cut into ½-inch pieces

¼ teaspoon red pepper flakes

3 cups chicken stock

2 cups water

1 pound fresh kale, stemmed and chopped

Coarsely ground black pepper

Fresh sea salt

1. Place a large Dutch oven on your gas or charcoal grill and prepare to medium heat. Leave the grill covered while heating, as it will add a faint smoky flavor to the skillet.

2. When the grill is ready, at about 400 degrees with the coals lightly covered with ash, add the olive oil into the Dutch oven, followed by the onion, garlic, and sausage pieces. Cook until the onion is brown and the sausage has browned, about 7 minutes. Remove the sausage from the pan and set aside.

3. Next, stir in the pepper flakes, chicken stock, and water and bring to a boil. Cook, uncovered, for about 20 minutes. Add in the kale and boil for about 5 more minutes until tender. Stir in the sausage and cook for about 2 more minutes.

4. Remove the Dutch oven from the grill and season with coarsely ground black pepper and fresh sea salt. Serve hot.

BIG TIP

Sausage can be a hard Paleo-friendly meat to come by. However, if you were to go to your local farmers' market or butcher, you should be able to find homemade sausage that works for your diet. It will be worth it, especially in this traditional Portuguese soup.

TURKEY VEGGIE STEW

SERVES: 8 / CALORIES: 293 / FAT: 14G / NET CARBS: 5G / PROTEIN: 22G

2 tablespoons olive oil

4 oz onion, chopped

2 cloves garlic, minced

1 teaspoon ground cumin

1 lb ground turkey

16-oz package frozen broccoli

3 cups chicken or vegetable stock

Salt and pepper to taste

1. In a large skillet over medium-high heat, cook the onion and garlic in the olive oil for 3 to 4 minutes. Sprinkle the cumin over the mix, and continue stirring and cooking another minute or so.

2. Add ground turkey and cook until meat is browned, about 5 minutes.

3. Put mixture into the slow cooker. Top with the frozen broccoli and the stock. Cover and cook on Low for 5 to 6 hours or on High for 2 to 3 hours. Season with salt and pepper to taste.

BIG TIP

This stew can be made more kid-friendly by making meatballs out of the turkey. Brown and cook them in the skillet before putting them in the slow cooker, and put the vegetables and broth around them. For more richness and fat, add in some heavy cream.

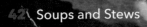

BOUILLABAISSE

SERVES: 8 / CALORIES: 170 / FAT: 6G / NET CARBS: 4G / PROTEIN: 26G

4 oz onion, chopped

2 cloves garlic, minced

1 stalk celery, fronds removed, finely chopped

1 red pepper, seeded and chopped

8 oz fish stock (or clam juice)

½ cup water

2 tablespoons extra virgin olive oil

1 tablespoon lemon zest

1 tablespoon fresh basil, chopped

1 tablespoon fresh parsley, chopped

1 teaspoon fresh oregano

1 teaspoon fresh thyme

1 bay leaf

1 lb firm white fish, cut into 1-inch pieces

¾ lb shelled, cleaned shrimp, tails removed

6.5-oz can chopped clams and the juice

8 oz cleaned, fresh crabmeat

Salt to taste

¼ cup fresh parsley, chopped

1. In a large bowl, combine onions, garlic, celery, red pepper, fish stock, water, olive oil, zest, spices, and bay leaf. Mix well. Put into slow cooker.

2. Cover and cook on Low for 4 to 5 hours or on High for 2 to 3 hours until base is hot and flavors are combined.

3. Stir in fish, shrimp, clams, and crab and cook for an additional 45 minutes to 1 hour or until fish is done (if cooking on High, reduce heat to Low). Remove bay leaf before serving. Season with salt to taste and stir in or garnish with parsley.

BIG TIP

This classic French fish "boil" is said to have originated in the seaside town of Marseilles in the south of France. The word itself has a fanciful attribution—bouille-besse, or the abbess' boil —in reference to a particular Abbesse in a convent there, as well as he more practical bouillon abaissé, meaning, "to reduce by evaporation." To increase the fat content of this dish, add in a tablespoon of butter to each serving; alternatively heavy cream can be added as well, depending on your preference.

CURRIED BROCCOLI SOUP

SERVES: 4 / CALORIES: 290 / FAT: 23G / NET CARBS: 7G / PROTEIN: 8G

4 tablespoons unsalted butter

2 oz onion, chopped

1 teaspoon curry powder

1 lb broccoli florets
(tough stems removed)

1 teaspoon baking soda

3 cups chicken broth

½ cup heavy cream

Salt and pepper to taste

1. In a skillet over medium heat, cook the onion in the butter until translucent, 2 to 3 minutes. Remove from heat and stir in the curry powder.

2. Transfer the onion mixture to the slow cooker. Add the broccoli. Stir the baking soda into the chicken broth until dissolved, and pour over broccoli. Cover and cook on Low for 6 hours or on High for 4 hours.

3. Add in the heavy cream, then use a hand-held emulsifier to puree the soup, or process it in batches in a blender. Season with salt and pepper.

BIG TIP

The addition of the baking soda will maintain the bright green color of the broccoli through the long cooking process. Heavy cream can be substituted with coconut cream if you prefer.

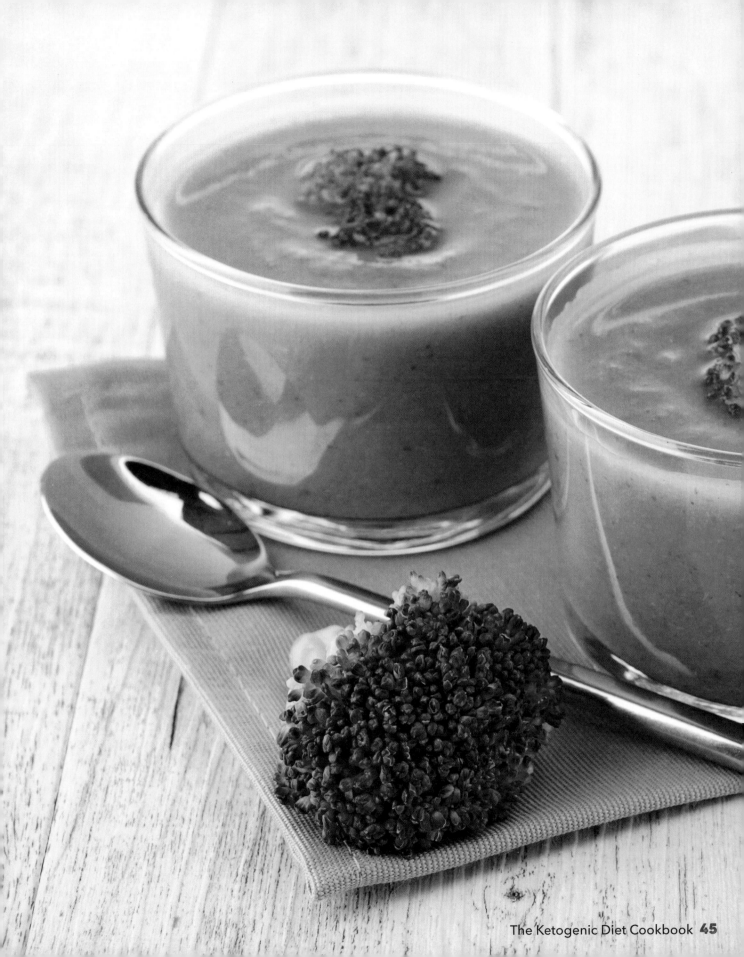

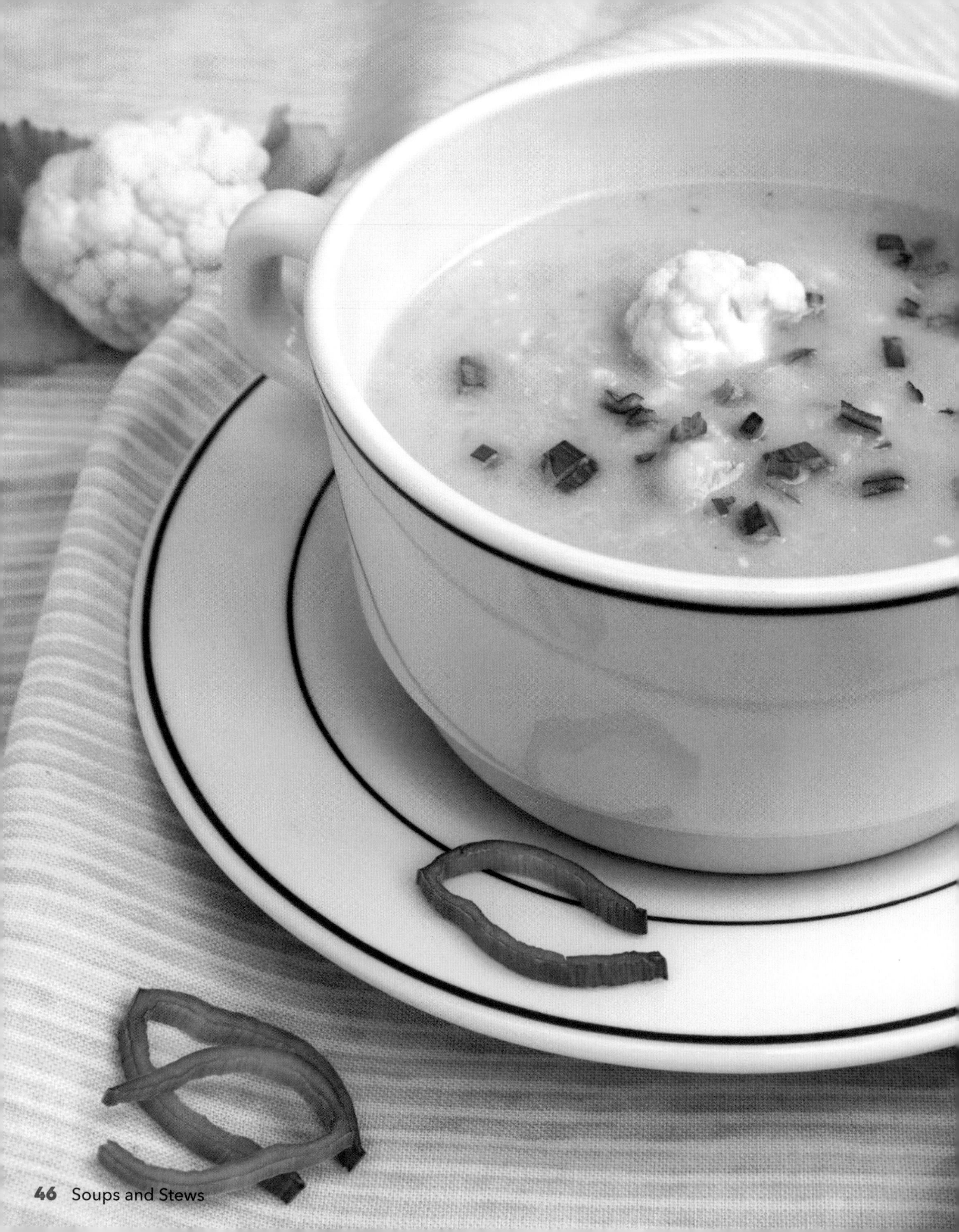

CREAMED CAULIFLOWER SOUP

SERVES: 4 / CALORIES: 387 / FAT: 4G / NET CARBS: 6G / PROTEIN: 7G

4 tablespoons extra virgin olive oil

4 oz onion, chopped

2 cloves garlic, minced

2 cups cauliflower, broken up into pieces, tough stem removed

2 cups chicken stock or broth

Salt and pepper to taste

8 oz heavy cream

Fresh tarragon leaves for garnish

1. In a skillet over medium-high heat, cook the onions and garlic in the olive oil until onions are translucent, about 5 minutes. Scrape mixture into the slow cooker.

2. Put the cauliflower pieces in the slow cooker, and pour the chicken stock on top. Cover and cook on Low for 6 to 8 hours or on High for 4 to 5 hours.

3. Puree the soup with an immersion blender or by batches in a blender. Season with salt and freshly ground pepper.

4. Transfer to a serving pot, and stir in the cream. When serving, garnish with 4 or 5 fresh tarragon leaves.

BIG TIP

Another option for a delicious and nutritious garnish is toasted almonds. To make them, preheat the oven to 350 degrees. On a cookie sheet, sprinkle sliced almonds. Cook them for 12 to 15 minutes, stirring every 4 to 5 minutes with a spatula until they are browned. Be careful not to overcook them. Transfer the cooked slices to a plate and allow to cool. Crumble or use whole.

MUSHROOM MADNESS

SERVES: 8 / CALORIES: 224 / FAT: 16G / NET CARBS: 6G / PROTEIN: 12G

6 pieces thick-cut bacon, diced

½ cup chopped yellow onion

½ teaspoon dried sage

¼ teaspoon cayenne pepper

½ lb fresh shitake mushrooms, stems removed, sliced

½ lb fresh cremini mushrooms, stems removed, sliced

1 lb fresh "baby" Portobello mushrooms, stems removed, sliced

1 oz dried porcini mushrooms

3½ cups chicken broth

8 oz heavy cream

Salt and pepper, to taste

1. In a skillet over medium heat, cook the bacon pieces, stirring frequently, until the bacon is crisp. Remove the meat from the pan, placing it on a paper towel over a plate to absorb some of the fat.

2. Add the onion to the skillet and cook it in the fat and bacon bits in the pan, stirring until the onion starts to wilt, about 2 minutes. Add the sage and cayenne, and stir. Remove from heat.

3. Put the sliced fresh mushrooms in the slow cooker. Add the bacon and onion mix. Add the dried porcini, and top with the broth. Stir to combine. Cover and cook on Low for 5 to 6 hours or on High for about 3 hours.

4. Stir in the heavy cream and season with salt and pepper to taste.

BIG TIP

The recipe calls for thick-cut bacon so that you get larger bacon pieces, but you can use any kind of bacon. Regular slices will yield smaller pieces. Smoked bacon will lend its flavor to the soup, as well, so if that's a flavor you like, try using that kind of bacon. You may want to skip the tamari if you choose smoked bacon.

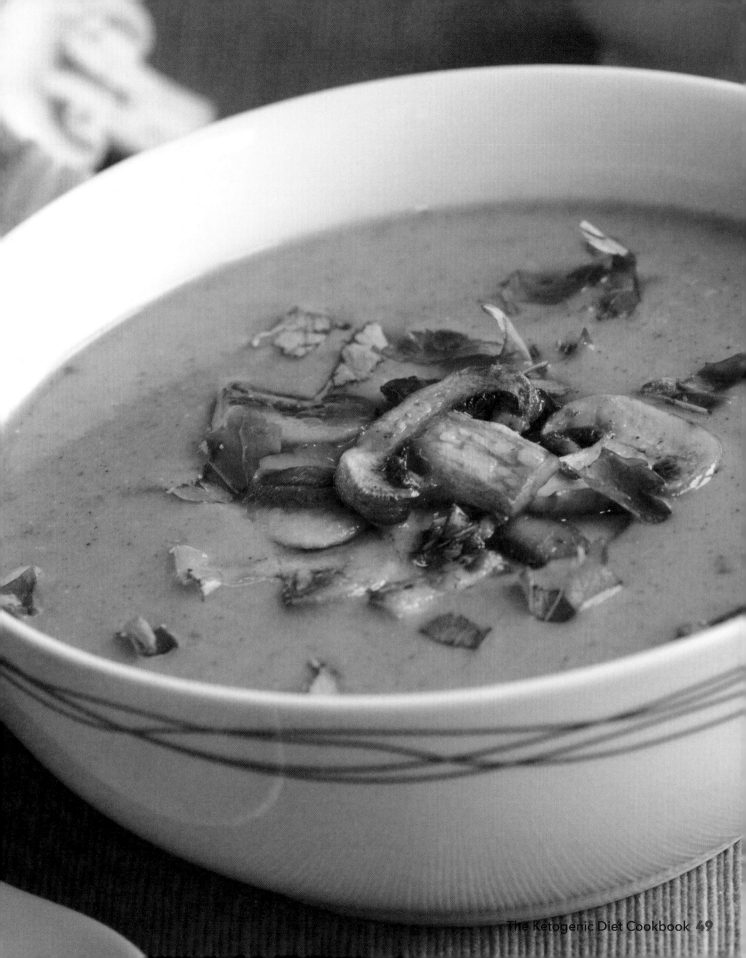

STARTERS & SIDES

On a diet, you never want to feel like you're missing out on good food, and on keto there's absolutely no reason to. Appetizers and sides are easily keto- customizable and a great way to build up to a stunning main course. A lot of these also work great as snacks, and can be made in advance and saved for those times you're feeling a bit peckish between meals.

The sides and starters in this section strike a great balance between meat and veggies. Salads, full of vibrant greens and fresh vegetables, barbecue staples, grills, skewers, sauces and rubs for you to toss the choicest ingredients through… everything here is designed to excite your palate and keep keto interesting. There are also a whole bunch of marinades that work great for meal prep – marinate your favorite cuts of meat and freeze them so you can pull them out on a day when you're not in the mood for an elaborate cook.

These appetizers are also great for when you're entertaining and your guests will never even know they're eating diet food. Can you imagine anyone turning down prosciutto-wrapped asparagus, deviled eggs or grilled calamari?

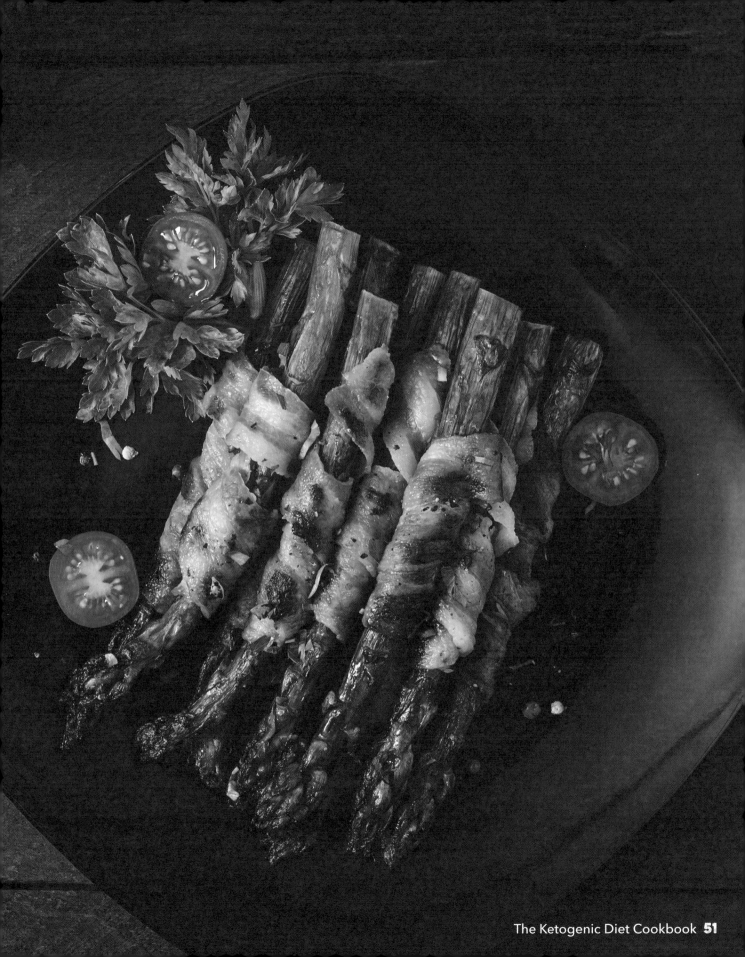

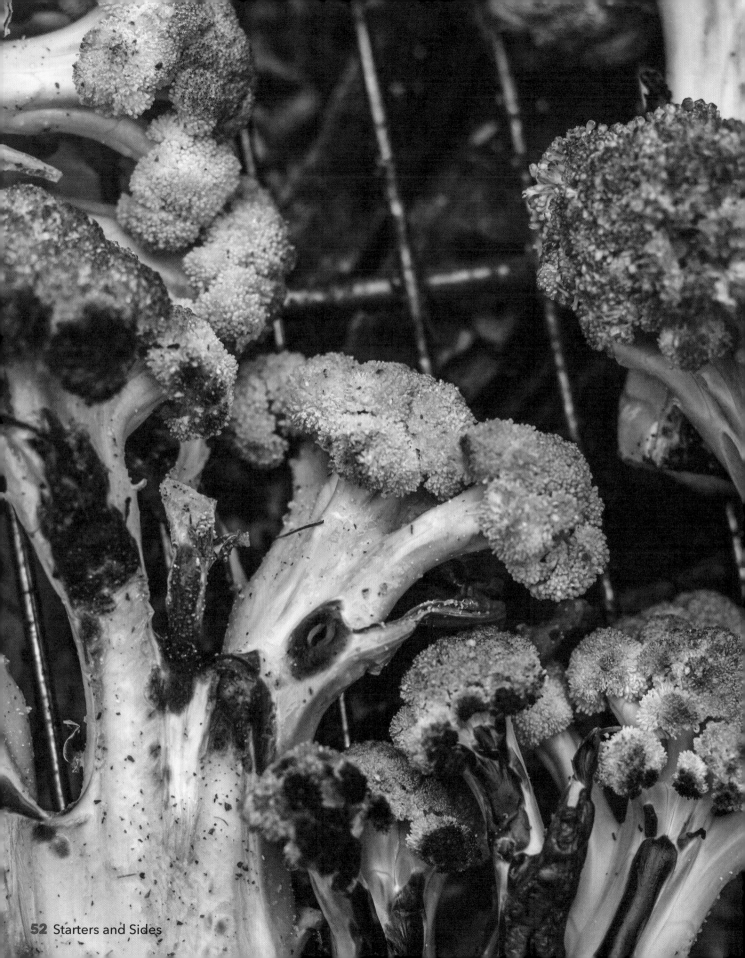

GRILLED BROCCOLI WITH LIME-BUTTER

SERVES: 4 / CALORIES: 309 / FAT: 26G / NET CARBS: 8G / PROTEIN: 4G

6 tablespoons clarified butter

¼ small lime, juiced

2 garlic cloves, finely chopped

½ teaspoon finely chopped cilantro

Coarsely ground black pepper

Fresh sea salt

16 oz broccoli florets

2 tablespoons olive oil

1. Prepare your gas or charcoal grill to medium heat.

2. Combine the clarified butter, lime juice, garlic, and cilantro into a small saucepan over extra-low heat and stir occasionally. Season with black pepper and sea salt.

3. When the grill is ready, about 400 degrees, brush the broccoli florets with olive oil and place on the grill. Cook until lightly charred, about 10 minutes, and then transfer to a medium bowl.

4. Remove the lime-butter from the burner and then mix with the broccoli florets. Serve warm.

BIG TIP

Grilled broccoli with lime-butter gives off a soft flavor that will never overpower its main course. It's great alongside pork or poultry.

MUSTARDY BRUSSEL SPROUTS

SERVES: 4 / CALORIES: 142 / FAT: 14G / NET CARBS: 2G / PROTEIN: 1G

1 lb Brussels sprouts

4 tablespoons extra virgin olive oil

1 teaspoon dry mustard

Pinch of sea salt

1. Wash and trim the Brussels sprouts, cutting off the coarsest part of the bottom and a layer or so of the leaves on the bottom. Cut the sprouts in half and put them in the slow cooker.

2. In a measuring cup, mix the olive oil with the dry mustard. Pour over the Brussels sprouts. Cover and cook on Low for 3 to 4 hours or on High for 2 to 3 hours. Before serving, add a pinch of sea salt.

BIG TIP

Mustard adds a wonderful tanginess to this recipe, but you can substitute other spices to get different flavors. For spicier sprouts, add some cayenne pepper or Asian chili sauce; for an Indian taste, add hints of curry or cumin.

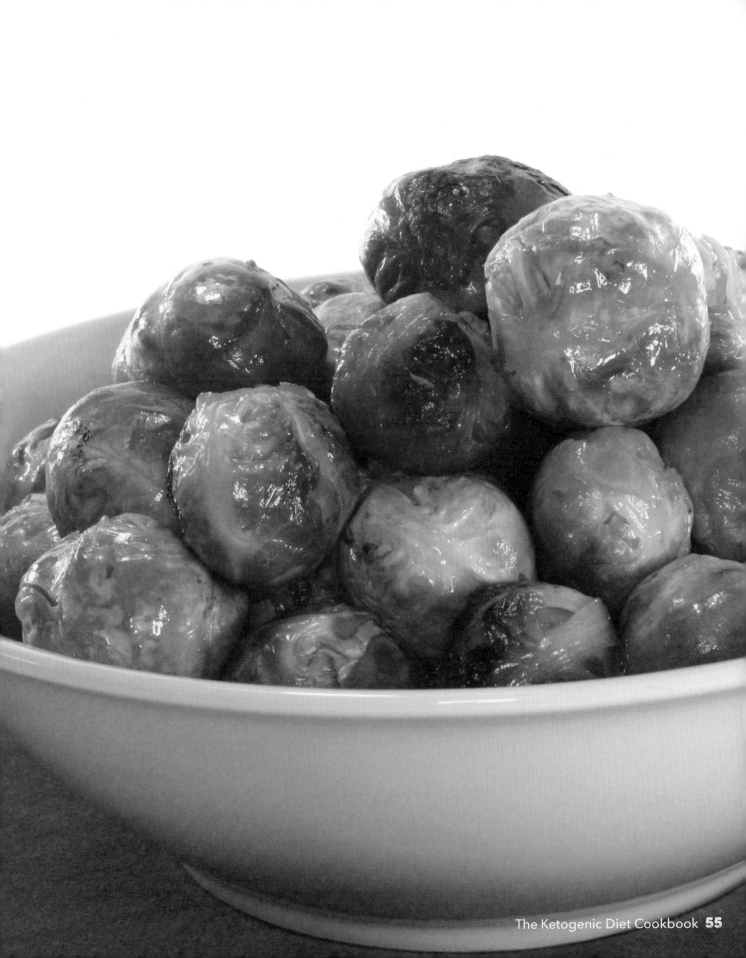

BACON DEVILED EGGS

SERVES: 6 / CALORIES: 514 / FAT: 50G / NET CARBS: 3G / PROTEIN: 2G

2 egg yolks, room temperature

¼ medium lemon, juiced

1 cup light olive oil

10 large eggs

6 thick strips of bacon

2 tablespoons Dijon mustard

2 tablespoons fresh parsley, finely chopped

Coarsely ground black pepper

Fresh sea salt

1 teaspoon paprika (optional)

3 chives, finely chopped (optional)

1. In a small food processor, add the 2 raw egg yolks and the lemon juice and puree for 30 seconds. Very gradually, add in the light olive oil until you reach a thick, mayonnaise-like consistency. It is extremely important to make sure that you add the light olive oil slowly to the processor, if you go too quickly, you will not reach the desired consistency.

2. Fill a medium saucepan with water. Carefully add the 10 eggs into the saucepan and then place the saucepan over medium heat. When the water reaches a boil, pull the eggs from the water and place under cool water. Let rest for a few minutes, and then peel back the shells.

3. Slice the eggs into halves. Using a fork, transfer the egg yolks from the eggs and place in a small bowl. Whisk in the Dijon mustard and parsley, and then season with coarsely ground black pepper and fresh sea salt. Set aside.

4. Place a medium frying pan over medium-high heat. Add the thick strips of bacon to the pan and cook until crispy, a few minutes on each side. (If you would like to add a smoked flavor to the bacon, consider smoking the bacon on the grill.) Transfer the bacon to a carving board and chop into bits. Whisk into the mixture.

5. Spoon the mixture from the small bowl back into the egg whites. If you would like, garnish with paprika and chopped chives. Serve chilled.

BIG TIP

These are perfect for football Sundays. The recipe is very straightforward and is easy to adapt for a larger gathering. Keep in mind that this is a foundational recipe and you can take and add any other flavors that come to mind!

HOUSE SALAD

SERVES: 6 / CALORIES: 308 / FAT: 30G / NET CARBS: 6G / PROTEIN: 3G

3 heads Romaine lettuce

1 small red onion, sliced into ¼-inch rings

10 Kalamata olives

10 green olives

4 plum tomatoes, stemmed and quartered

6 pepperoncini peppers

2 garlic cloves, minced

¼ cup red wine vinegar

¾ cup olive oil

Coarsely ground black pepper

Fresh sea salt

1. Rinse the heads of Romaine lettuce and dry them thoroughly. In a medium bowl, combine the lettuce, red onion, Kalamata olives, green olives, tomatoes, and pepperoncini peppers and then set in refrigerator.

2. In a small jar, whisk together the minced garlic, red wine vinegar, and olive oil, and then season with coarsely ground black pepper and fresh sea salt. Chill in refrigerator for 15 minutes.

3. Remove the salad and the vinaigrette from the refrigerator and mix together. Serve immediately.

BIG TIP

This basic, hearty salad is a good complement to a large steak or pork chop. For something different, pair this with a side of Grilled Dijon Veggies.

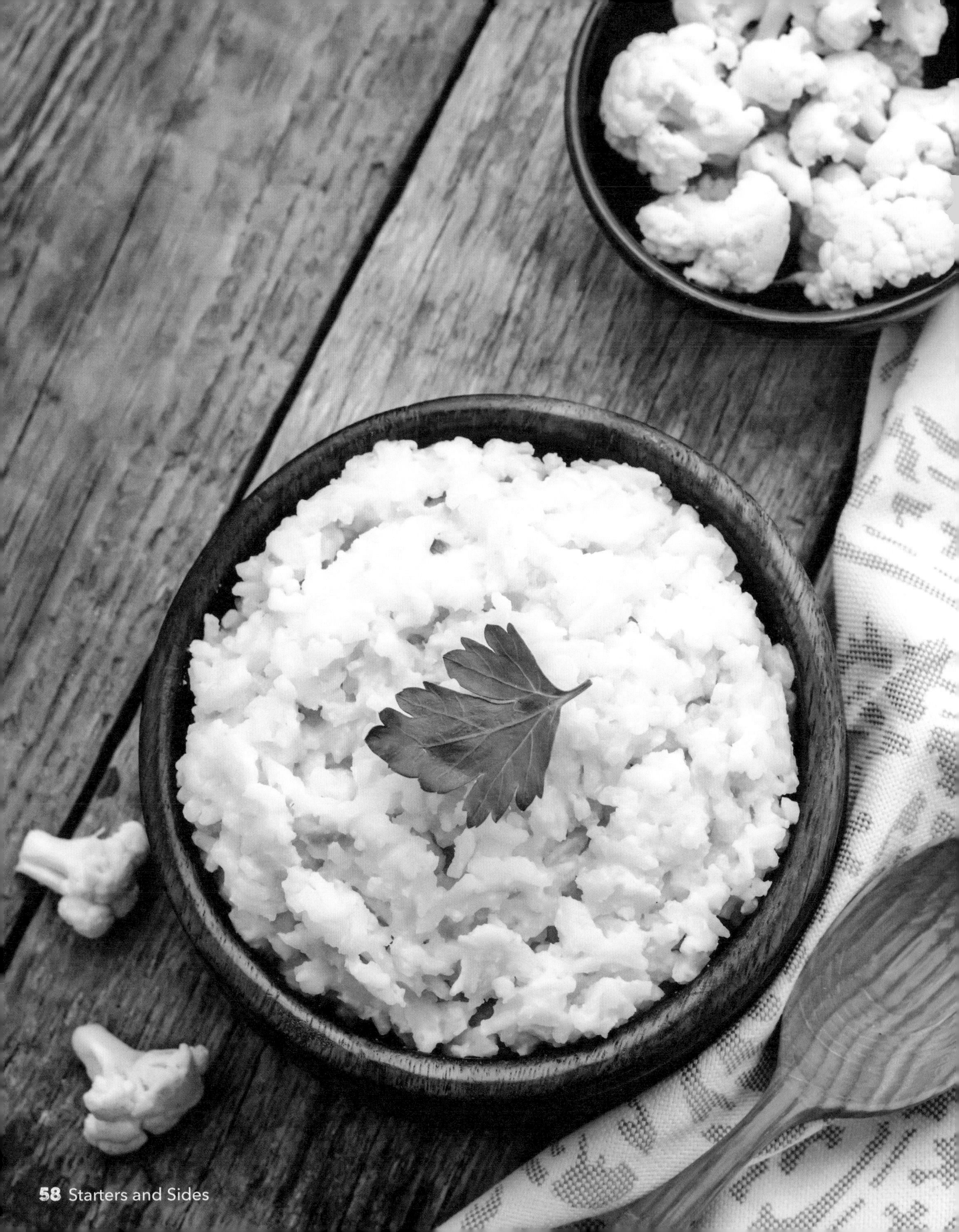

CAULIFLOWER RICE

SERVES: 2 / CALORIES: 345 / FAT: 28G / NET CARBS: 11G / PROTEIN: 8G

1 large head of cauliflower

4 tablespoons extra virgin oil

Salt and pepper, to taste

1. In a food processor, pulse the cauliflower until it reduces to the size of grains.

2. In a skillet over medium heat, heat olive oil and cook your cauliflower rice for 3-5 minutes, covered. Sprinkle with salt and pepper to taste.

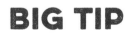

BIG TIP

A simple rice substitute that doesn't sacrifice flavor.

CAULIFLOWER STEAKS

SERVES: 4 / CALORIES: 231 / FAT: 19G / NET CARBS: 7G / PROTEIN: 7G

1 large cauliflower

¼ cup olive oil

1 tablespoon lemon juice

2 cloves garlic, minced

2 oz shredded pepper jack cheese

1 pinch red pepper flakes, to taste

Salt and pepper, to taste

1. Begin by slicing the cauliflower lengthwise through the core into four pieces—these will become your "steaks." Preheat your grill to medium-high heat.

2. Mix the olive oil, lemon juice, garlic, pepper flakes, salt and pepper with a whisk.

3. Place the steaks into foil large enough to surround the steaks and seal them into a packet. Generously brush the mixture on both sides of the cauliflower. Seal the packet and place on the grill. Cook for about 8 minutes, or until tender. Flip the steaks about halfway through.

4. Once it is slightly browned, remove from heat, sprinkle shredded pepper jack over the tops and serve.

BIG TIP

Steak isn't just for meat-eaters. Try this gluten-free option using cauliflower from the garden, pair with some red wine and enjoy.

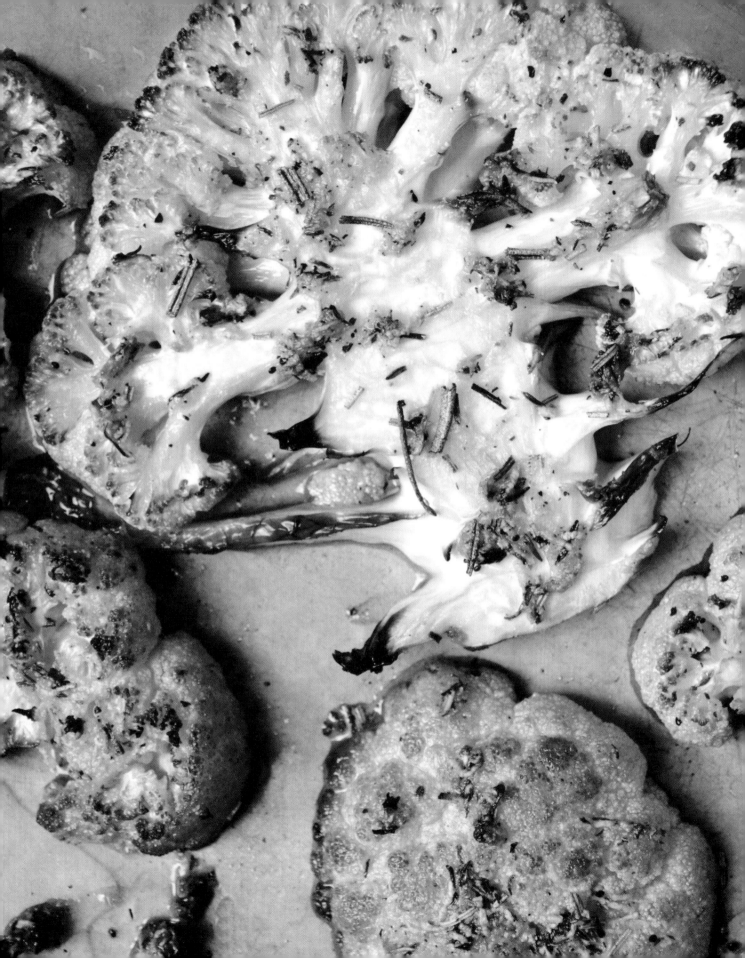

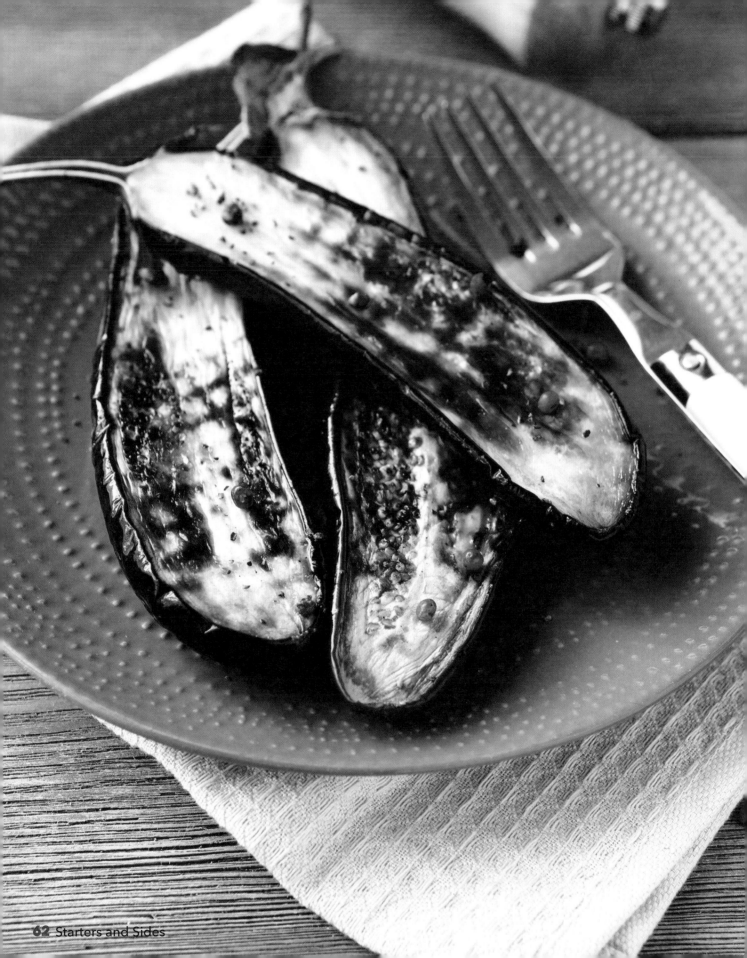

CAJUN GRILLED EGGPLANT

SERVES: 4 / CALORIES: 162 / FAT: 15G / NET CARBS: 5G / PROTEIN: 2G

1 cup brown rice

2 small eggplants, cut into ½-inch slices (approximately 32 oz in total weight)

¼ cup olive oil

2 tablespoons lime juice

1 tablespoon Cajun seasoning

1. Cook brown rice according to package instructions and let stand.

2. In a small bowl, mix together olive oil, lime juice and Cajun seasoning. Brush this mixture over both sides of the eggplant and let them sit for about 5 minutes.

3. Preheat your grill to medium heat and cook the slices until they become tender. This should take about 4-5 minutes per side. Remove from heat and serve over rice.

BIG TIP

Serve this with 1 pound of skinless, boneless chicken breast. Grill over medium heat for 5-6 minutes, until thoroughly cooked through. Add a dollop of butter over for extra flavor and fat.

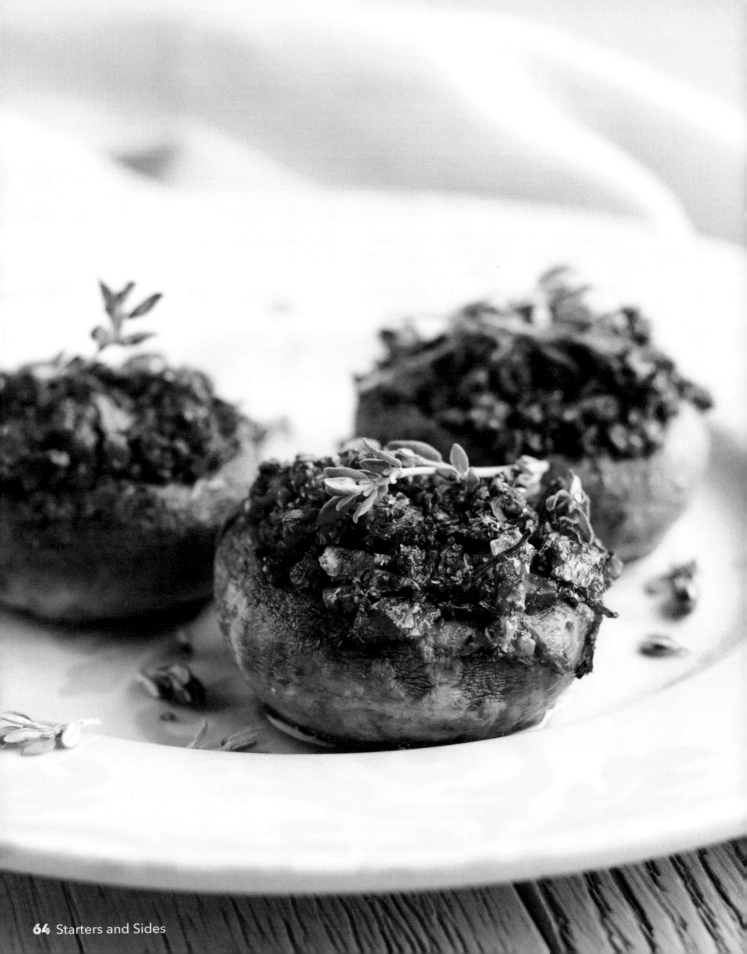

CHORIZO-STUFFED MUSHROOMS

SERVES: 8 / CALORIES: 86 / FAT: 8G / NET CARBS: 3G / PROTEIN: 2G

1 Spanish chorizo, casing removed (approximately 4 oz)

14 white mushrooms, stemmed

¼ cup, plus 2 tablespoons olive oil

2 oz white onion, finely chopped

¼ cup chicken broth

1 small bunch parsley, finely chopped

Coarsely ground black pepper

Fresh sea salt

1. Prepare your gas or charcoal grill to medium heat. Leave a cast-iron skillet on the grill while heating so that it develops a faint, smoky flavor.

2. While waiting, add the chorizo into a food processor and puree into a thick paste. Remove and set aside.

3. When the grill is ready, at about 350 to 400 degrees with the coals lightly covered with ash, brush the mushroom caps with the 2 tablespoons of olive oil.

Next, place the mushroom tops on the grill and cook for about 2 minutes until the tops have browned. Remove from grill and place on a baking sheet.

4. Next, add the remaining ¼ cup of olive oil to the cast-iron skillet, followed by the onion. Cook until the onion is translucent, about 2 minutes, and then stir in the pureed chorizo. Continue to cook until the chorizo is lightly browned, about 3 minutes, and then add in the chicken broth and parsley. Cook for only a minute or so longer, and then remove from heat.

5. Using a spoon, add the chorizo mixture into the mushroom caps. Move the baking sheet to a cool side of the grill and cook for about 15 minutes until the chorizo has browned. Remove from the grill, season with coarsely ground black pepper and fresh sea salt, and serve hot.

BIG TIP

Note: Macros will vary depending on the brand and size of the chorizo used. Add some cheddar cheese to up the fat macros of the dish and also for a delicious cheesy stuffed mushroom.

GRILLED MUSHROOM SKEWERS

SERVES: 4 / CALORIES: 137 / FAT: 11G / NET CARBS: 5G / PROTEIN: 3G

½ pound medium white mushrooms

2 oz bell peppers, cut into chunks

2 oz onion, cut into chunks

¼ cup melted butter

½ teaspoon dill weed

½ teaspoon garlic salt

1. Thread mushrooms, peppers and onions onto 4 skewers.

2. In a small bowl, combine butter, dill and garlic salt. Brush this mixture over the skewers.

3. Preheat grill to medium-high heat and grill skewers for 10–15 minutes, turning occasionally. Remove from heat and serve.

BIG TIP

Mushroom kebabs are great because they soak up the marinade extremely well. The bell peppers ensure that this skewer is equal parts savory and refreshing.

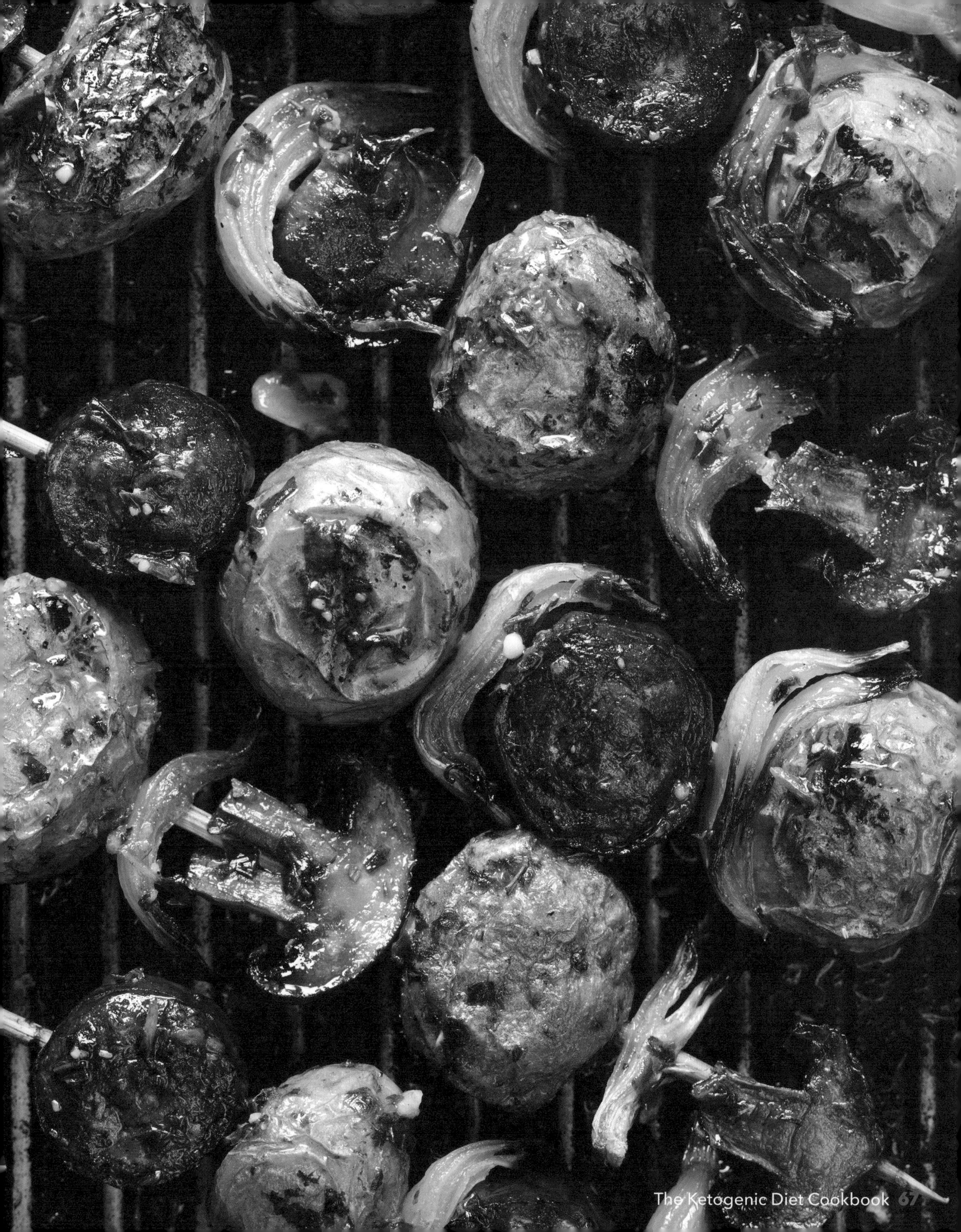

CAJUN GREEN BEANS

SERVES: 4 / CALORIES: 140 / FAT: 12G / NET CARBS: 5G / PROTEIN: 2G

1 pound green beans, trimmed

½ teaspoon Cajun seasoning

4 tablespoons butter

1. Prepare a large piece of foil to create a foil packet. Place the green beans on the foil and sprinkle the seasoning over them, along with butter. Fold the edges around the beans and crimp the edges to seal the packet tightly.

2. Preheat your grill to medium heat and place the packet on the grill seam side up. Cook for about 20 minutes, rotating the packet about 10 minutes in. Remove from heat when beans are tender and serve.

BIG TIP

Add Meat: Remove the packets after about 15 minutes and wrap the green beans in half slices of bacon. Place them back in the foil packets or directly on the grill and cook until the beans are tender and the bacon is crisp.

JALAPENOS FILLED WITH SAUSAGE AND DICED TOMATOES

SERVES: 6 / CALORIES: 257 / FAT: 19G / NET CARBS: 7G / PROTEIN: 7G

2 tablespoons olive oil

1 pound pork sausage

2 garlic cloves, minced

¼ small red onion, minced

3 tablespoons minced red bell pepper

8 cherry tomatoes, minced

12 jalapeno peppers, halved and seeded

Coarsely ground black pepper

Fresh sea salt

1. Prepare your gas or charcoal grill to medium heat. Leave a cast-iron skillet on the grill while heating so that it develops a faint, smoky flavor.

2. When the grill is ready, at about 350 to 400 degrees with the coals lightly covered with ash, heat the olive oil in the skillet and then add the pork sausage. Cook until the sausage is no longer pink but evenly brown.

3. When the sausage is near complete, add the garlic and onion and cook until translucent, about 2 to 3 minutes. Stir in the red bell peppers and the cherry tomatoes and cook for another 2 minutes or so. Transfer the sausage stuffing from the grill and let rest.

4. Arrange the halves of the jalapeño peppers evenly on a baking sheet. Using a spoon, add the sausage mixture into the cavities of the peppers. Transfer to the grill and cook, covered, for about 20 minutes until lightly browned. Remove from the grill, season with pepper and salt, and serve immediately.

BIG TIP

Grilled stuffed jalapeños are simple and quick to prepare. Although the jalapeños are considered a hot pepper, when you seed and grill them, their heat is toned down and softer. For the sausage, if you are looking to save some time, pick up organic pork sausage (from a local butcher, if possible). It never fails!

GRILLED DIJON VEGGIES

SERVES: 6 / CALORIES: 188 / FAT: 17G / NET CARBS: 6G / PROTEIN: 2G

¼ cup olive oil

2 tablespoons red wine vinegar

½ teaspoon dried oregano

1 teaspoon Dijon mustard

1 clove garlic, minced

Pinch of salt and pepper

2 medium zucchini,
cut into ¼-inch rounds

1 medium summer squash,
cut into ¼-inch rounds

1 small red onion, cut into wedges

2 oz bell pepper, cut into 2-inch strips

4 oz mushrooms

6 cherry tomatoes

4 tablespoons butter

1. In a small bowl, combine the oil, red wine vinegar, dried oregano, Dijon and garlic and mix well.

2. Place the vegetables in a large, resealable bag and toss to coat with the dressing. Let this stand for about 15 minutes in the refrigerator.

3. Preheat your grill to medium heat and place the vegetables on the grill rack. Cook until they become tender, about 10–12 minutes. Remove from heat, finish with the butter and serve.

BIG TIP

If you love mustard, I recommend increasing the amount of Dijon you include in this recipe. Its sharp flavor profile pairs nicely with any fresh vegetable.

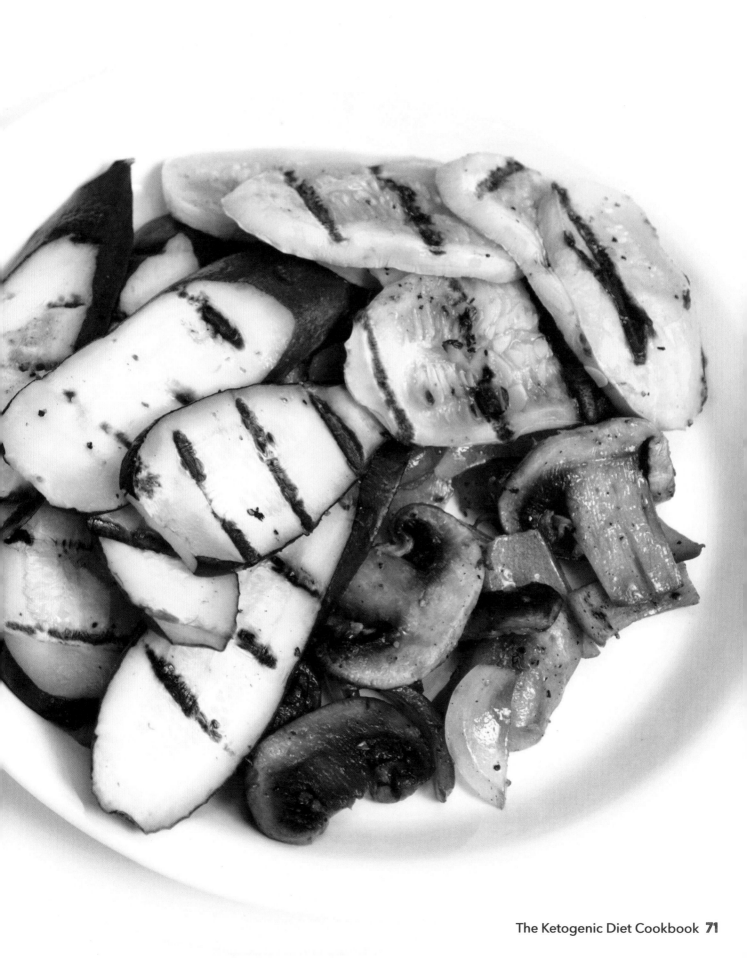

ASPARAGUS WITH PROSCIUTTO

SERVES: 6 / CALORIES: 297 / FAT: 24G / NET CARBS: 2G / PROTEIN: 18G

1 lb asparagus

1 lb prosciutto, sliced very thin

1 tablespoon clarified butter or ghee, melted

1. Wash and dry asparagus spears, trimming off tough bottoms by about an inch.

2. Wrap each spear in a slice of prosciutto, and lay the spears gently and carefully in the slow cooker. Drizzle the spears with the melted butter. Cover and cook on Low for about 2 hours or on High for about 1 hour, until spears are tender.

3. Turn heat to High and cook for an additional 15 to 20 minutes with the lid propped open with the handle of a wooden spoon to allow steam to escape. This will dry-crisp the pancetta somewhat.

BIG TIP

While thin spears are usually more desirable for quick cooking when steaming asparagus, for this recipe it is preferable to select fatter spears so there is more inside the wrap of prosciutto.

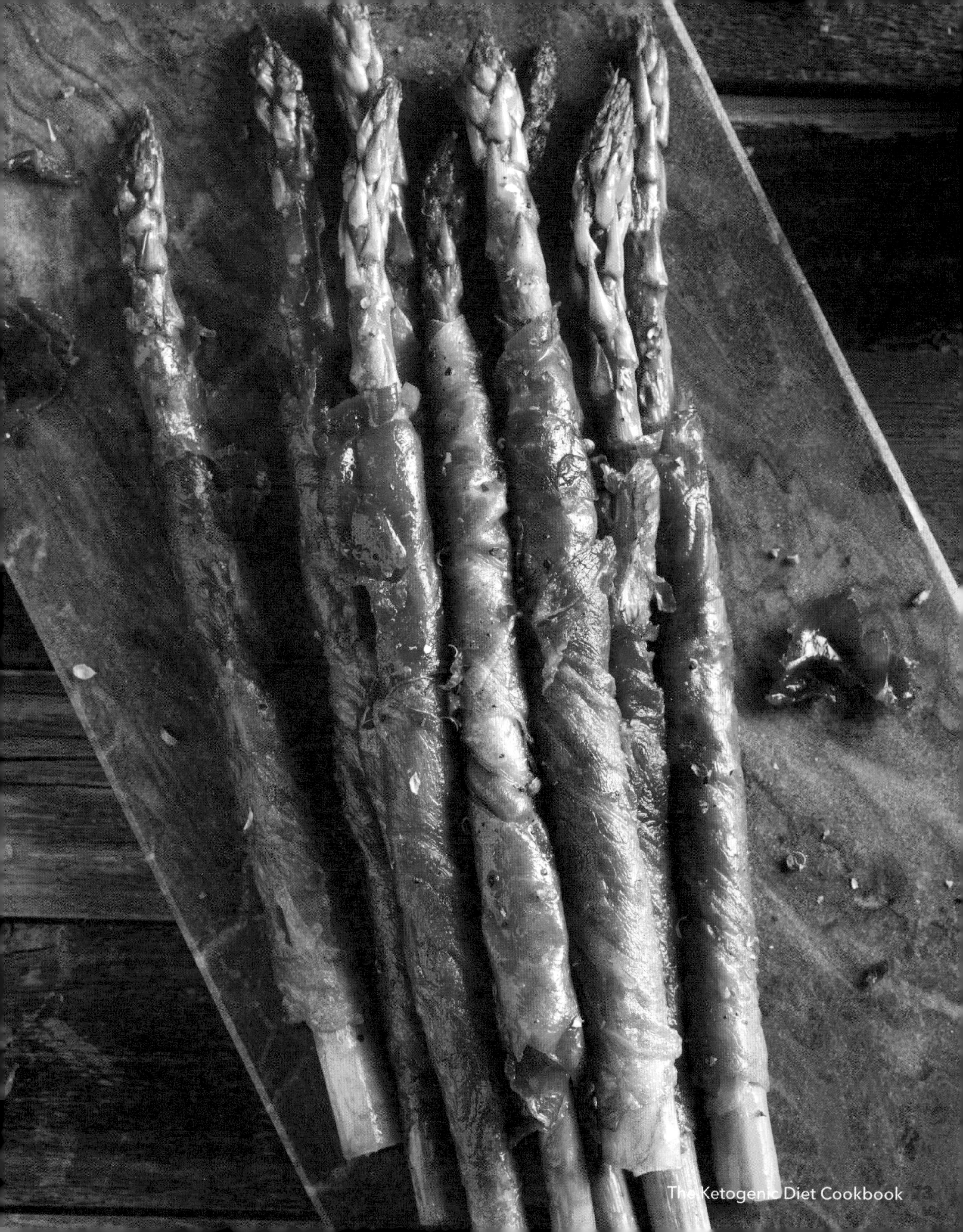

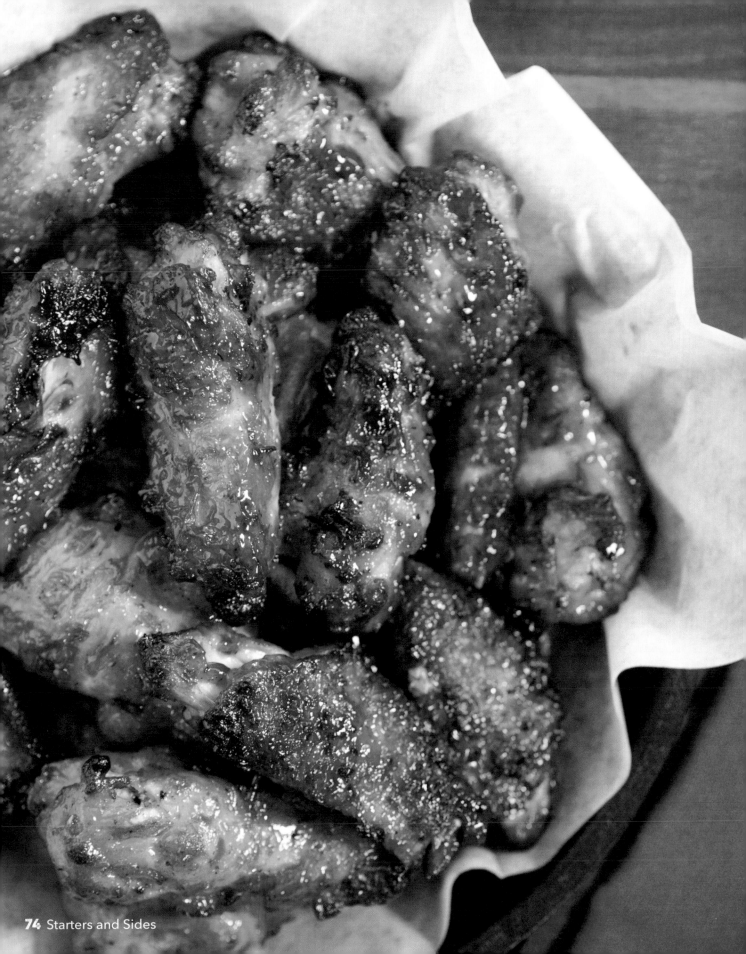

CLASSIC BUFFALO WINGS

SERVES: 6 / CALORIES: 319 / FAT: 20G / NET CARBS: 7G / PROTEIN: 25G

2 pounds chicken wings, split

2 tablespoons clarified butter

3 garlic cloves, minced

¼ teaspoon cayenne

¼ teaspoon paprika

2 teaspoons Sriracha sauce

1 head celery, stalks cut into 3-inch pieces

1. Place the chicken wings on a roasting pan and put in the refrigerator. Let rest for at least 2 hours so that the skin on the wings tightens, promoting a crisp wing.

2. One hour before grilling, add the woodchips into a bowl of water and let soak.

3. A half hour before grilling, prepare your gas or charcoal grill to high heat.

4. In a small saucepan, add the clarified butter over medium heat. When hot, add the garlic and cook until golden—about 2 minutes. Next, mix in all of the remaining ingredients and bring to a simmer of medium heat. Simmer for about 3 minutes and then remove from heat and place in a large bowl.

5. Remove the chicken wings from the refrigerator and toss with the buffalo sauce in the large bowl.

6. When the grill is ready, at about 450 degrees with the coals lightly covered with ash, scatter the woodchips over the coals and then place the chicken wings on the grill with a good amount of space between them. Cover the grill and cook for about 2 to 3 minutes on each side, frequently basting each wing with the remaining buffalo sauce. Remove from grill when the skin is crispy.

7. Place on a large serving platter and serve warm alongside celery.

BIG TIP

Perfect for a Sunday with the boys, this dish never gets old. For this recipe, I decided to add a smoky flavor to the wings by adding a couple cups of pre-soaked hickory or oak woodchips to the coals. This style is optional, though I strongly recommend it.

GRILLED CALAMARI

SERVES: 6 / CALORIES: 224 / FAT: 11G / NET CARBS: 6G / PROTEIN: 24G

1 lemon, juiced

¼ cup olive oil

2 garlic cloves, finely chopped

2 sprigs fresh oregano,
leaves removed

Coarsely ground black pepper

Fresh sea salt

2 pounds fresh squid, tentacles
separated from bodies

1. Combine the lemon juice, olive oil, garlic, and oregano in a large bowl. Season with coarsely ground black pepper and fresh sea salt. Add the squid to the bowl and let marinate for 1 to 2 hours.

2. Prepare your gas or charcoal grill to medium-high heat. Leave a cast-iron skillet on the grill while heating so that it develops a faint, smoky flavor.

3. When the grill is ready, at about 400 degrees with the coals lightly covered with ash, place the squid tentacles and rings in the skillet and cook until opaque, about 3 to 4 minutes. When finished, transfer the squid to a large carving board and let stand at room temperature for 5 minutes before serving.

BIG TIP

To hit your fat macros, add a tablespoon of butter to each serving.

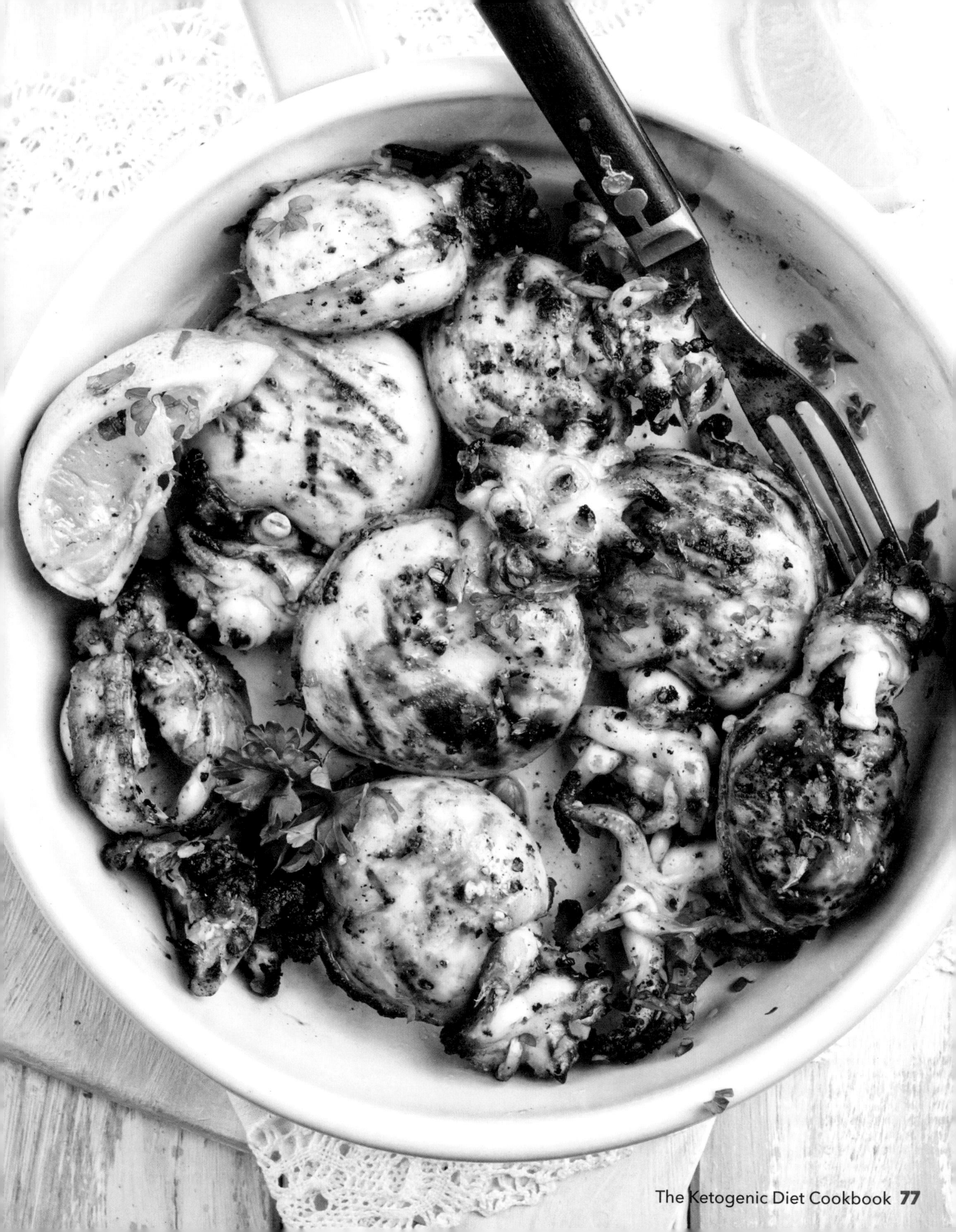

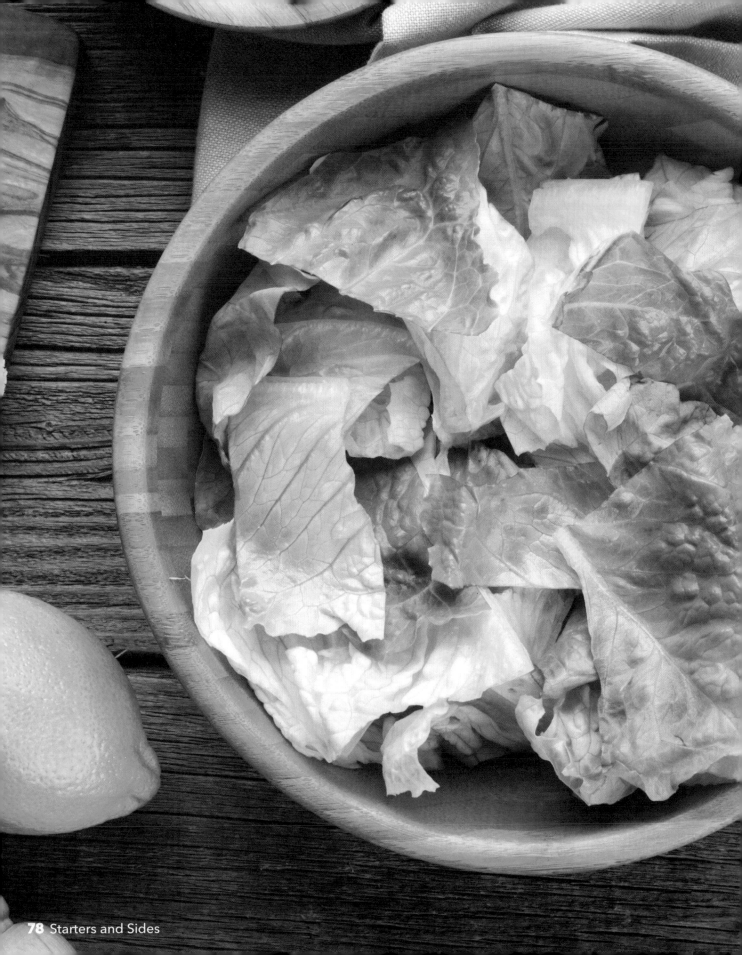

CLASSIC CAESAR SALAD

SERVES: 6 / CALORIES: 205 / FAT: 20G / NET CARBS: 3G / PROTEIN: 4G

3 heads Romaine lettuce

2 garlic cloves, minced

½ small lemon, juiced

1 large egg

4 anchovy filets

1 teaspoon Dijon mustard

½ cup olive oil

Coarsely ground black pepper

Fresh sea salt

1. Rinse the heads of Romaine lettuce and then dry thoroughly. Place in refrigerator and set aside.

2. In a small bowl, whisk the minced garlic, lemon juice, and egg until blended. Whisk in the anchovy filets and Dijon mustard until the anchovies have been completely incorporated into the dressing.

3. Gradually whisk in the olive oil and then season with coarsely ground black pepper and sea salt. Place the dressing in the refrigerator for about 15 minutes and then pour over the chilled Romaine lettuce. Serve immediately.

BIG TIP

Top this salad with grilled chicken or smoked bacon.

FRISÉE SALAD

WITH MAPLE-SMOKED BACON AND HARDBOILED EGGS

SERVES: 6 / CALORIES: 152 / FAT: 12G / NET CARBS: 3G / PROTEIN: 7G

---

1 pound frisée

3 large eggs

8 thick slices of bacon,

2 tablespoons white wine vinegar

2 tablespoons red wine vinegar

1 teaspoon Dijon mustard

2 tablespoons olive oil

Coarsely ground black pepper

Fresh sea salt

1. One hour before grilling, soak the maple woodchips in water.

2. Next, place a large cast-iron skillet on your gas or charcoal grill and prepare to medium heat. Leave the grill covered while heating, as it will add a faint smoky flavor to the skillet.

3. While waiting, rinse the frisée and dry thoroughly. Place the frisée in a medium bowl and store it in the refrigerator.

4. Next, fill a medium saucepan with water and place over medium-heat. Bring to a boil and then add the eggs and remove from heat. Cover the saucepan and let the eggs rest in the hot water for about 10 to 14 minutes. Remove from water and let cool in the refrigerator.

5. When the grill is ready, at about 400 degrees with the coals lightly covered with ash, throw the wood chips over the coals and cover the grill. When the grill is smoking, add the bacon into the cast-iron skillet, close the grill's lid, and cook until crispy, about 4 minutes. Transfer to a plate covered with paper towels and set aside.

6. In a small bowl, whisk together the white wine vinegar, red wine vinegar, Dijon mustard, and olive oil and then set aside.

7. Remove the eggs from the refrigerator and then peel off their shells. Slice the eggs in half and add over the frisée salad. Drizzle the vinaigrette onto the frisée and then top with the bacon bits. Season the eggs with the coarsely ground black pepper and fresh sea salt and then serve the salad immediately.

BIG TIP

I serve this salad as a main course, sometimes with a side of grilled veggies with Walnuts and typically with a glass of white wine.

GREEN BEAN AND ARUGULA SALAD

SERVES: 4 / CALORIES: 106 / FAT: 11G / NET CARBS: 3G / PROTEIN: 1G

1 bunch fresh green beans

3 tablespoons extra virgin olive oil

1 bunch arugula

1 red bell pepper, chopped

2 tablespoons balsamic vinegar

Pinch of salt and pepper

1. Clean and trim green beans, then coat them with olive oil. Add salt and pepper to taste.

2. Preheat your grill to medium heat and coat the grates with oil. Spread the beans over the grate. Cover and cook for 15-20 minutes, making sure to rotate.

3. Once the beans are crispy and cooked through, remove them and toss with arugula, vinegar and chopped bell pepper, and more extra virgin olive oil.

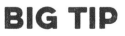

BIG TIP

ADD MEAT! Prepare 1¼ pounds of skirt steak by seasoning with salt and pepper. Grill this for 5 minutes per side, or until it reaches desired doneness. Serve in slices over the salad.

ARUGULA SALAD
WITH TARRAGON-SHALLOT VINAIGRETTE

SERVES: 6 / CALORIES: 184 / FAT: 19G / NET CARBS: 3G / PROTEIN: 2G

1 pound of Arugula lettuce, stemmed

1 shallot, minced

5 stalks tarragon, minced

¼ small lemon, juiced

1 teaspoon Dijon mustard

½ cup olive oil

3 tablespoons red wine vinegar

Coarsely ground black pepper

Fresh sea salt

1. Rinse the arugula and then dry thoroughly. Place in refrigerator and set aside.

2. In a small bowl, whisk together the shallot, tarragon, lemon juice, and Dijon mustard, and then slowly add in the olive oil and red wine vinegar.

3. Season with coarsely ground black pepper and fresh sea salt, and then pour over the arugula. Serve immediately.

BIG TIP

This hearty salad is quick to make and full of flavor. Serve it with white wine.

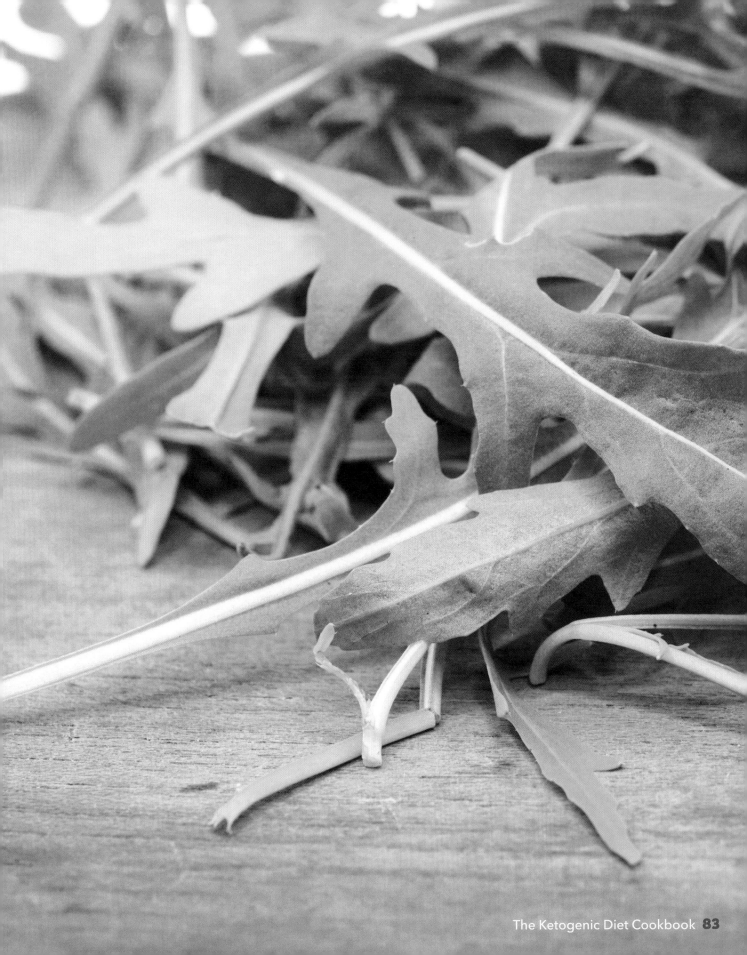

LEMON ASPARAGUS SALAD

SERVES: 4 / CALORIES: 235 / FAT: 21G / NET CARBS: 3G / PROTEIN: 7G

¼ cup olive oil

¼ cup lemon juice

1 bunch asparagus spears

⅛ cup Parmesan cheese, grated

6 cups spring greens salad mix

1 tablespoon Parmesan-seasoned almond slices

1 cup cherry tomatoes

1 pinch salt and pepper

1. Preheat grill to low heat. In a bowl, combine asparagus, lemon juice and oil and toss to coat asparagus.

2. Grill the asparagus spears for about 5 minutes, making sure to turn while they're cooking. Remove from heat once tender.

3. In a large serving bowl, combine the spring greens, Parmesan cheese, almond slices, cherry tomatoes, salt and pepper.

4. Slice the asparagus into bite-sized pieces and add them to the salad with the lemon juice and olive oil. Toss the salad and serve.

BIG TIP

This salad is heavily asparagus-based, but it's just as easy to substitute the spears out for any other vegetable you prefer.

GRILLED ROMAINE SALAD

SERVES: 4 / CALORIES: 99 / FAT: 8G / NET CARBS: 3G / PROTEIN: 3G

2 tablespoons extra virgin

1 head romaine lettuce, cut in half lengthwise

1 tablespoon steak seasoning

2 tablespoons lemon juice

2 tablespoons Parmesan cheese, for sprinkling

1. Toss romaine lettuce with olive oil and season with steak seasoning.

2. Preheat your grill for medium heat. Oil the grates lightly to prevent sticking. Place the lettuce directly on the grill cut side down and cook for about 5 minutes. The lettuce is done cooking when it becomes slightly wilted and lightly charred.

3. Remove from heat, drizzle with lemon juice and sprinkle Parmesan cheese on top. Serve and enjoy!

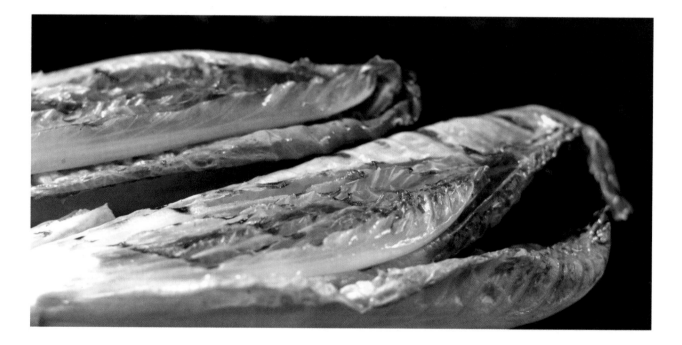

BIG TIP

Grilled romaine may feel a bit uninspired, but the common leafy green provides a nice crunch alongside the steak seasoning flavors. Serve this with grains or meat.

EGGPLANT SALAD

SERVES: 3 / CALORIES: 169 / FAT: 14G / NET CARBS: 6G / PROTEIN: 2G

1 large eggplant

1 medium tomato, diced

1½ teaspoon red wine vinegar

½ teaspoon oregano

2 garlic cloves, diced

3 tablespoons olive oil

3 tablespoons parsley, chopped

Pinch of salt and pepper, to taste

1. Preheat grill to medium-high heat. Prick the eggplant with a fork, place on the grill and cook for about 15 minutes, covered. Cook until skin is soft, turning eggplant occasionally. Remove from heat and let cool.

2. Once the eggplant is cool, scoop out the insides and chop. Place this in a bowl and toss with diced tomatoes, vinegar, oregano, garlic and salt.

3. Add in the oil, parsley and pepper. Mix together and serve.

BIG TIP

In my opinion, the insides of an eggplant make the perfect salad topping. But if you disagree, try substituting your favorite squash instead.

The Ketogenic Diet Cookbook

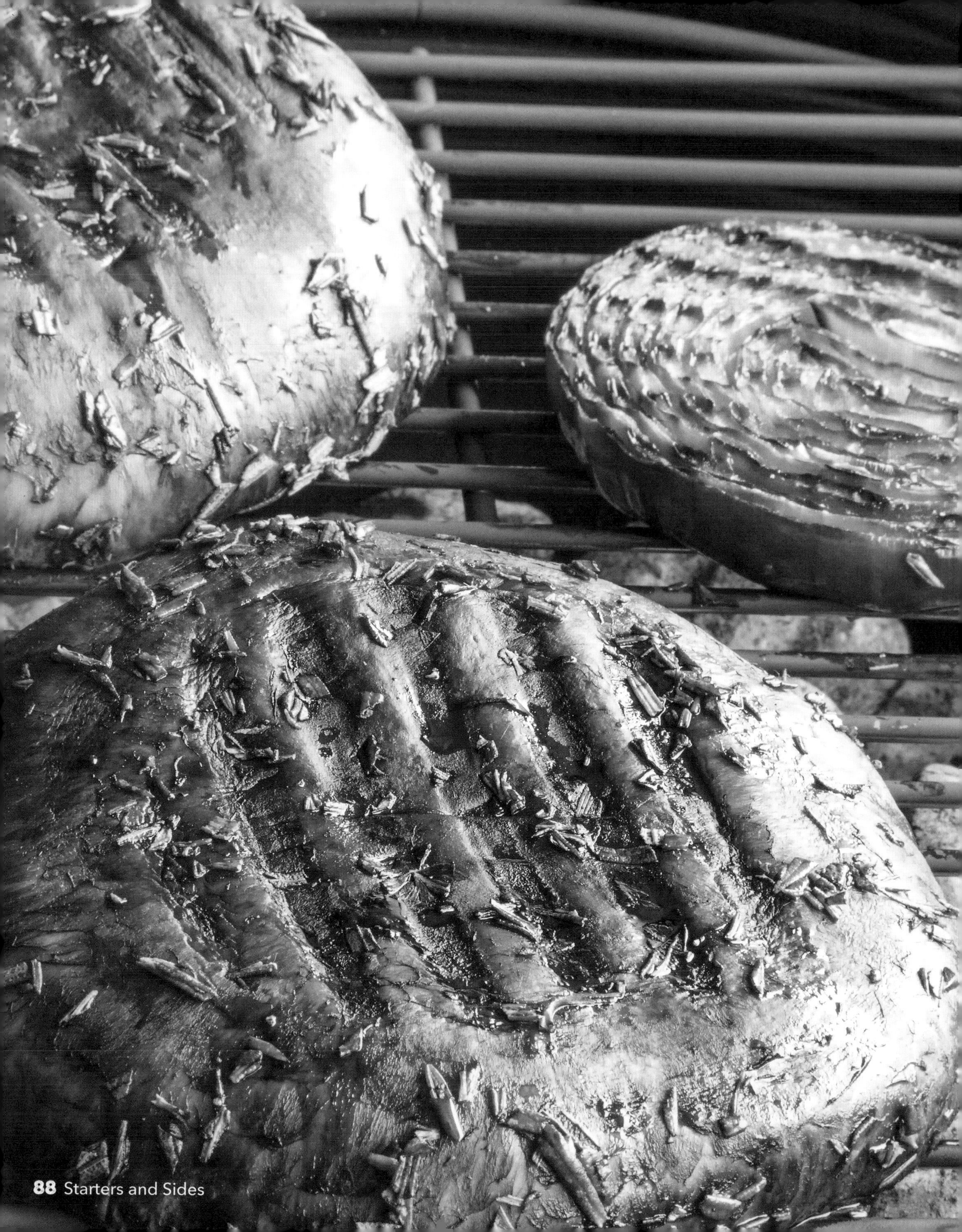

GRILLED PORTOBELLO SALAD

SERVES: 4 / CALORIES: 160 / FAT: 11G / NET CARBS: 6G / PROTEIN: 8G

4 large portobello mushrooms

7 oz grape tomatoes, halved

3 ounces fresh mozzarella, cubed

6 fresh basil leaves, torn

2 tablespoons extra virgin

2 cloves garlic, minced

2 cups salad greens

Salt and pepper, to taste

1. In a small bowl, mix together tomatoes, mozzarella, basil leaves, olive oil, garlic, salt and pepper. Place to the side and let sit.

2. Remove the stems and gills from mushrooms and lightly brush with oil.

3. Grill the mushrooms covered for 6–8 minutes per side, or until the caps become tender.

4. Remove from heat and dice the mushrooms.

5. In a large bowl toss the tomato mixture, salad greens and diced mushrooms, and serve.

BIG TIP

When you introduce the grill, every salad improves, and no recipe exemplifies that concept better than one with grilled portobellos. Enjoy this Italian-style salad in any season.

BASIL PESTO

SERVES: 6 / CALORIES: 228 / FAT: 22G / NET CARBS: 2G / PROTEIN: 7G

⅓ cup, plus 2 teaspoons extra-virgin olive oil

⅓ cup pine nuts

3 cups fresh basil leaves

2 garlic cloves

¼ cup Parmesan cheese, freshly grated

Coarsely ground black pepper

Fresh sea salt

1. Add 2 teaspoons of the extra-virgin olive oil to a small frying pan and place on the stovetop over medium heat. When hot, add the pine nuts and toast for a minute or two until golden, not browned. Remove from the heat and transfer to a small cup.

2. In a small food processor, pulse the pine nuts, basil leaves, and garlic into a thick paste. Next, slowly incorporate the remaining extra-virgin olive oil into the pesto, until you reach your desired consistency.

3. Using a spatula, remove the pesto from the processor and place in a medium bowl. With a spoon, mix in the Parmesan cheese and then season with the coarsely ground black pepper and fresh sea salt. Serve at room temperature, or lightly chilled.

BIG TIP

Pesto is rooted in herbs and pine nuts—two of the most versatile flavors.

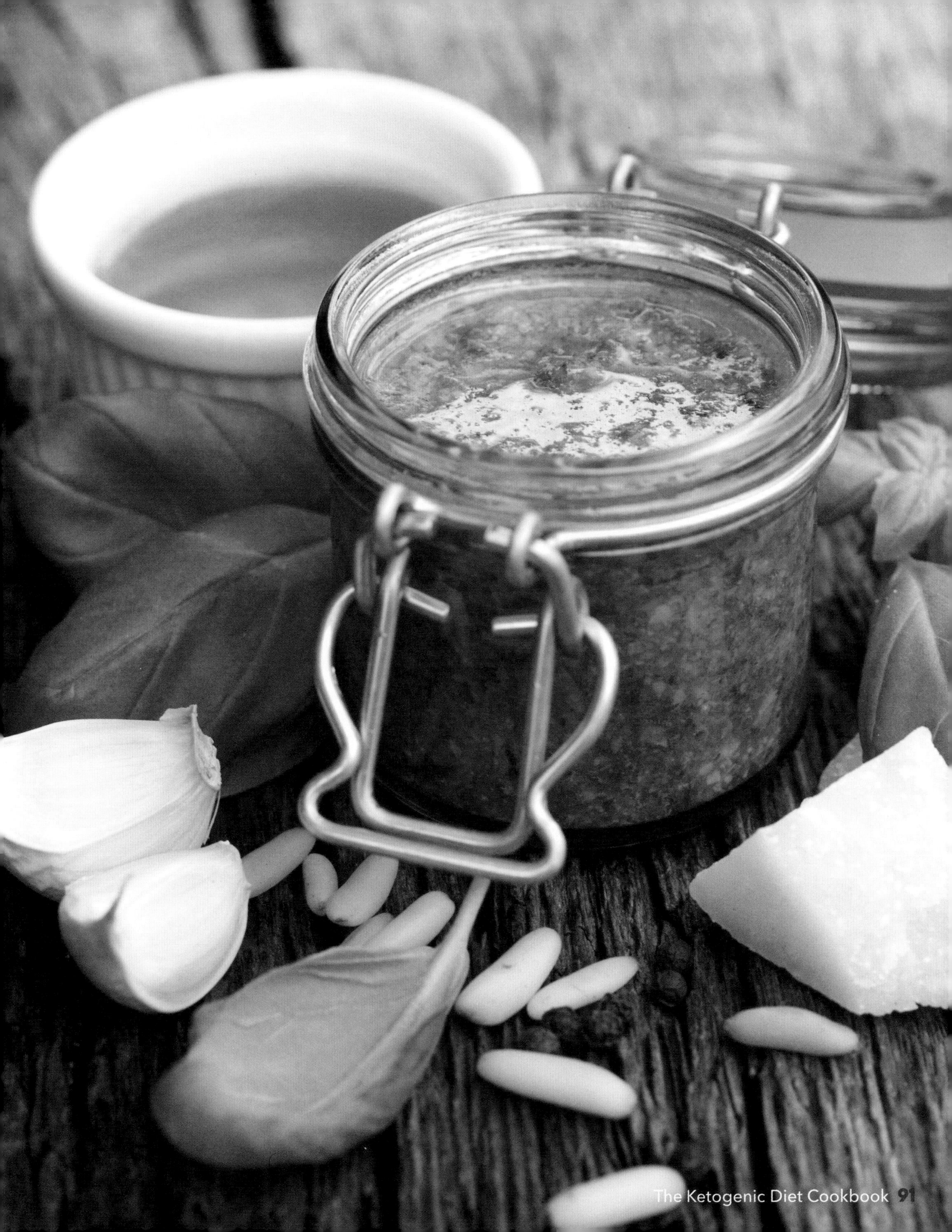

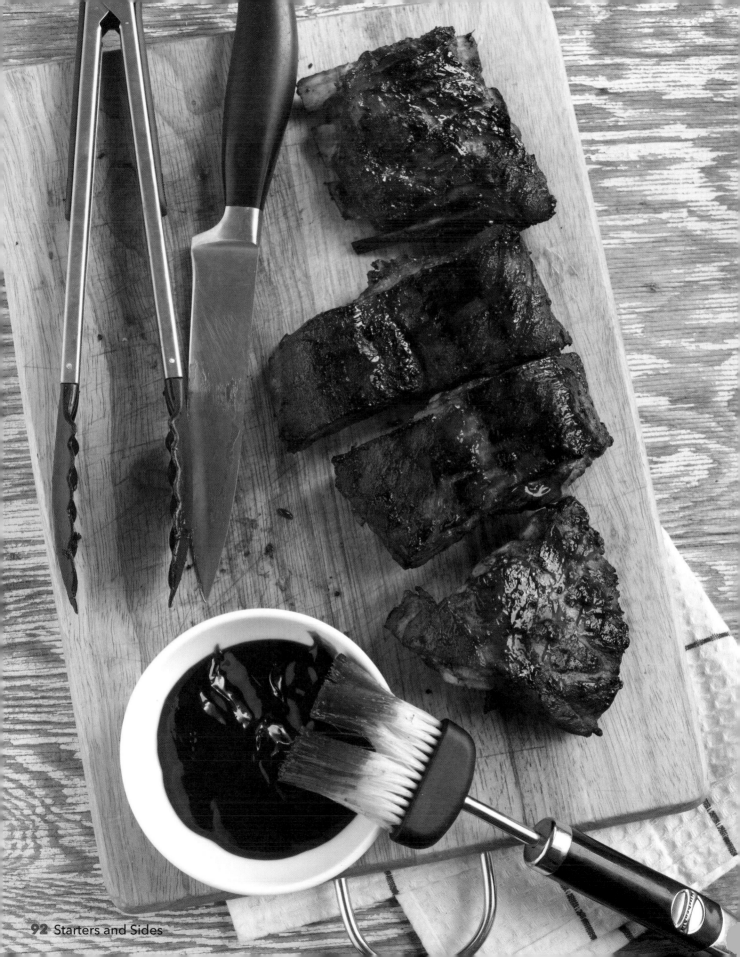

SMOKED SOUTHERN BBQ SAUCE

SERVES: 12 / CALORIES: 63 / FAT: 4G / NET CARBS: 4G / PROTEIN: 1G

4 tablespoons butter

2 garlic cloves, finely chopped

1 medium white onion, finely chopped

16 oz tomatoes, chopped finely

¼ cup tomato paste

¼ cup white wine vinegar

¼ cup balsamic vinegar

2 tablespoons Dijon mustard

1 medium lime, juiced

2 tablespoons ginger, finely chopped

1 teaspoon smoked paprika

½ teaspoon ground cinnamon

2 dried chipotle peppers, finely chopped

1 habanero pepper, seeded and finely chopped (optional)

1 cup water

Coarsely ground black pepper

Fresh sea salt

1. An hour before grilling, add the woodchips into a bowl of water and let soak.

2. Prepare your gas or charcoal grill to medium-high heat.

3. While waiting for the grill to heat up, place a small frying pan over medium heat and, when hot, add the butter, garlic and onion and cook until the garlic has browned and the onion is translucent. Remove and set aside.

4. Transfer the cooked garlic and onion into a food processor, followed by the tomatoes and tomato paste. Puree into a thick paste, and then add the remaining ingredients to the food processor and blend thorough. Transfer the sauce into to a medium saucepan and set alongside the grill.

5. When the grill is ready, about 400 to 450 degrees with the coals lightly covered with ash, drain 1 cup of the woodchips and spread over the coals or pour in the smoker box. Place the medium saucepan on the grill and then bring the sauce to a boil with the grill's lid covered, aligning the air vent away from the woodchips so that their smoke rolls around the sauce before escaping. Let the sauce cook for about 30 to 45 minutes, every 20 minutes adding another cup of drained woodchips, until it has reduced to about 2 cups.

6. Remove the sauce from the heat and serve warm. The sauce can be kept refrigerated for up to 2 weeks.

BIG TIP

This sauce is filled with intense spice and goes great when served on or alongside barbecued beef and pork dishes. The habanero pepper is optional in this recipe and should be used only for those who like their BBQ sauces hot!

MEAT SAUCE

SERVES: 10 / CALORIES: 209 / FAT: 13G / NET CARBS: 4G / PROTEIN: 19G

2 tablespoons extra-virgin olive oil

2 tablespoons butter

1 medium onion, chopped fine

1 green bell pepper, seeds and rib removed, chopped fine

8 oz button mushrooms, rinsed and sliced thick

1 lb ground beef

1 lb ground turkey

2 14.5-oz cans diced tomatoes, undrained

3 cloves garlic, minced

2 teaspoon dried oregano

1 tablespoon dried basil

1 teaspoon red pepper flakes

Salt and pepper to taste

1. In a large skillet over medium-high heat, add the olive oil, butter, onion, pepper, and mushrooms. Cook, stirring, for about 3 minutes, and put in the bottom of the slow cooker.

2. In the same skillet, brown the ground meats together over medium heat, being careful not to cook too long. The meat should be slightly pink. Put it in the slow cooker on top of the vegetables.

3. Add the tomatoes, garlic, oregano, basil, and red pepper flakes. Stir to combine. Cover and cook on Low for 4 to 6 hours or on High for about 2 hours. Season with salt and pepper.

BIG TIP

While you can't eat regular pasta on a low-carb diet, you can make a delightful bowl of spaghetti squash upon which to serve this sauce. You can also slice long zucchini with a mandoline to make "noodles." When you have been on the low-carb diet for a while, you can experiment with low-carb pastas, but they must be eaten only on occasion. Lots of other foods are great with spaghetti sauce!

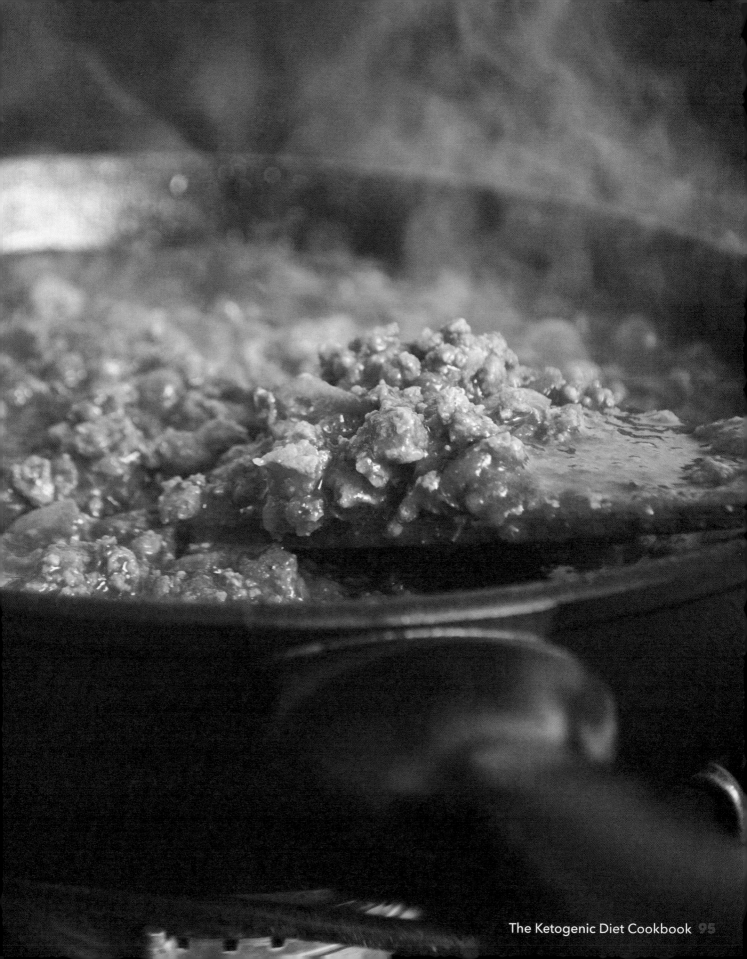

BASIC AU JUS

SERVES: 8 / CALORIES: 72 / FAT: 6G / NET CARBS: 50G / PROTEIN: 1G

½ cup dry red wine

2 cups beef broth

4 tablespoons unsalted butter

Coarsely ground black pepper

Fresh sea salt

1. To begin, strain rib roast drippings through a fine sieve. Then, pass the strained juiced through a fat separator (a simple spoon will do). Add the juices to the roasting pan and set over medium-high heat; note that you may need to use two burners.

2. Add the wine to your roasting pan, along with 2 cups of beef broth (note the 1:2 ratio here between the red wine and beef broth). Do not add a stock to your au jus; always a broth.

3. With the roasting pan placed over medium-high heat, bring your juices to a boil and then reduce until you have about 1 to 1½ cups of au jus. Stir the au jus occasionally, scraping off the browned bits from the bottom so that they naturally are incorporated into the au jus.

4. Remove the roasting pan from the heat and season with the coarsely ground black pepper and fresh sea salt.

BIG TIP

Note: If you can find a sugar free wine or a wine with less sugar the carb content will be lower, you can also add more butter to increase the fat macros.

RUSTIC PEPPER DRY RUB

SERVES: 4 / CALORIES: 11 / FAT: 0G / NET CARBS: 2G / PROTEIN: 0G

---

2 garlic cloves, minced

2 teaspoons fresh thyme, finely chopped

2 teaspoons fresh sea salt

1½ teaspoons coarsely ground black pepper

1½ teaspoons coarsely ground white pepper

1 teaspoon coarsely ground red pepper

1 teaspoon sweet paprika

½ teaspoon onion powder

1. In a small bowl, stir together all the ingredients and then apply generously to the rib roast, massaging the rub into the marbled section of the roast so that the spices become properly ingrained in the meat.

—— BIG TIP ——

A little spicy, I recommend using this rub on a summer evening when you decide to cook the roast with a charcoal pit technique.

BARBECUE RUB

SERVES: 4-6 / CALORIES: 9 / FAT: 0G / NET CARBS: 1G / PROTEIN: 0G

1 teaspoon cumin

1 teaspoon paprika

1 teaspoon garlic powder

1 teaspoon onion powder

1 teaspoon chili powder

1 teaspoon salt

¼ teaspoon ground black pepper

1. Mix ingredients together in a small bowl!

BIG TIP

A simple rub can make all the difference when barbecuing something, whether it be half a zucchini or 10 ounces of steak. This one is particularly nice because it works with all diets.

MEMPHIS RUB

SERVES: 4 / CALORIES: 28 / FAT: 0G / NET CARBS: 2G / PROTEIN: 1G

2 tablespoons coarsely ground black pepper

1 tablespoon smoked paprika

2 teaspoons yellow mustard seeds

2 teaspoons fresh sea salt

1 teaspoon ground cumin

1 teaspoon dried oregano

1 teaspoon garlic powder

½ teaspoon cayenne pepper

1. In a small bowl, thoroughly combine all the ingredients and store in an air-tight container at room temperature for up to 1 month.

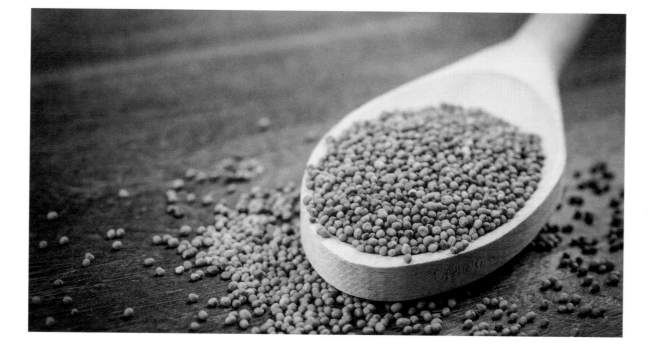

BIG TIP

This very strong rub is perfect when you are grilling up some beef or pork ribs. Knead it firmly into the meaty parts of the ribs so that the meat is filled with succulent flavor.

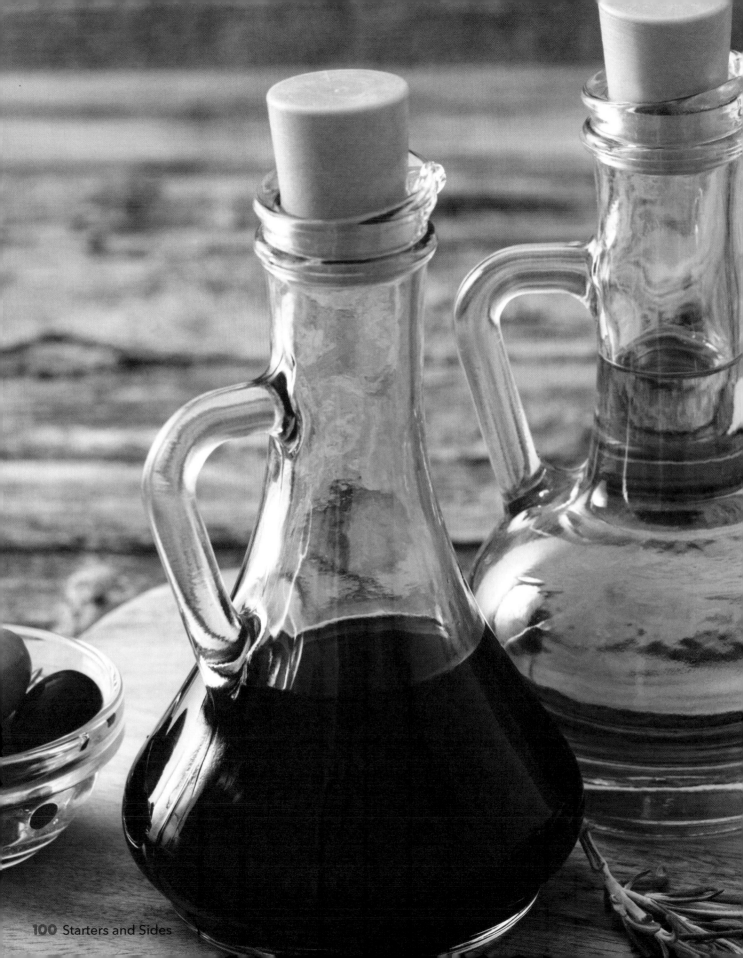

BALSAMIC MARINADE

SERVES: 4 / CALORIES: 126 / FAT: 14G / NET CARBS: 1G / PROTEIN: 0G

4 tablespoons extra-virgin olive oil

2 tablespoons balsamic vinegar

2 tablespoons lemon juice

1 tablespoon Dijon mustard

2 cloves garlic, minced

Pinch of salt and pepper

1. Mix the ingredients in a small bowl and use as a marinade on just about everything!

BIG TIP

Acidic and just a little sweet, balsamic flavors pair so well with vegetables—especially if they've had time to marinate prior to being grilled or tossed. Try this with zucchini, tomatoes, eggplant or any salad you've thrown together.

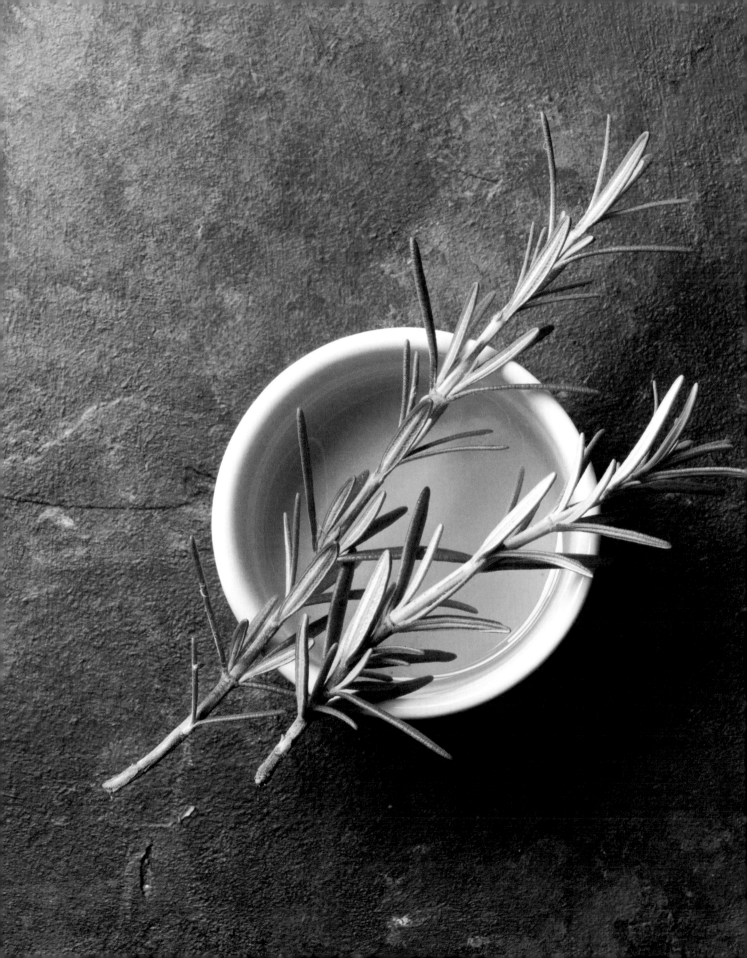

ROSEMARY-INFUSED OLIVE OIL

SERVES: 8 / CALORIES: 242 / FAT: 28G / NET CARBS: 0G / PROTEIN: 0G

6 large sprigs fresh rosemary

1 cup extra- virgin olive oil

Coarsely ground black pepper

Fresh sea salt

1. In a small saucepan, combine the rosemary and extra-virgin olive oil and place on the stovetop with the heat off. Set the heat to medium-low and let the olive oil heat, but do not let it reach a boil. When hot, turn the heat off and let the rosemary infuse into the olive oil for 1 to 2 hours.

2. Strain the oil into a jar and keep at room temperature or in the refrigerator. Store for 2 or 4 months, respectively.

BIG TIP

The soft rosemary flavors always go well around with a rib roast and its sides. It's extremely simple to infuse olive oil, and I usually double this recipe so that when I prepare my rib roast I'll rub it with the rosemary-infused olive oil.

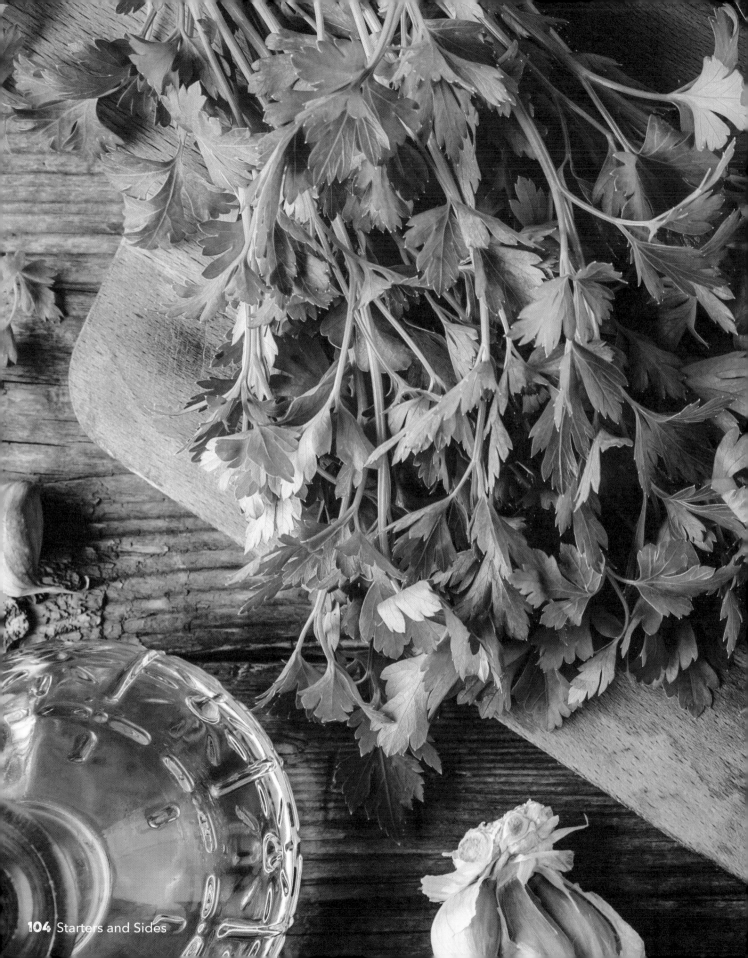

LEMON-PARSLEY MARINADE

SERVES: 4 / CALORIES: 106 / FAT: 113G / NET CARBS: 10G / PROTEIN: 2G

2 medium lemons, juiced

2 garlic cloves, finely chopped

¼ cup fresh parsley, finely chopped

¼ cup fresh basil, finely chopped

1 tablespoon red bell pepper, finely chopped

1 tablespoon coarsely ground black pepper

2 teaspoons fresh sea salt

½ cup extra-virgin olive oil

1. In a medium bowl, combine all the ingredients and let rest for 15 minutes so the flavors can spread throughout the marinade.

2. Add the rib roast to the marinade. Transfer to the refrigerator and let marinate for about 4 hours. If the marinade does not fully cover the meat, turn the meat halfway through the marinating process so that all areas of the meat receive equal amounts of the marinade.

BIG TIP

Use this marinade for quick, last-minute meals, especially seafood dishes, as both the lemon and parsley flavors are mild when grilled. Pair with white wine.

MAINS

On the keto diet, people seem to think that mains are just big hunks of meat drowned in butter and oil – which it can be, if that's what you fancy – but it's so much more than that. There's no reason your main course can't be an incredible tasting dish, well balanced and full of flavor, and it's surprising how much "regular" food lends itself to keto – think pork vindaloo, chicken parm, turkey meatballs (with zucchini spaghetti!). Hankering after an unhealthy pizza? Sub in eggplant slices or portobello mushrooms for a delicious veggie "pizza" or go a step further and make a cauliflower crust.

Here you'll find recipes for every keto mood. No time to cook an elaborate meal on a weekday? Seafood mains are quick to cook and chock-full of Omega-3 fats and healthy protein and will come together in minutes. Eating alone? Some grilled basil chicken breast is just the ticket. For those long weekends when you're putting together a week's worth of meals, there are great slow cooker recipes that you can throw together overnight and wake up to a delicious dish for the next day. And if you'd really just like a big hunk of meat, a porterhouse with chimichurri sauce or a crown roast of beef is easy, and achievable.

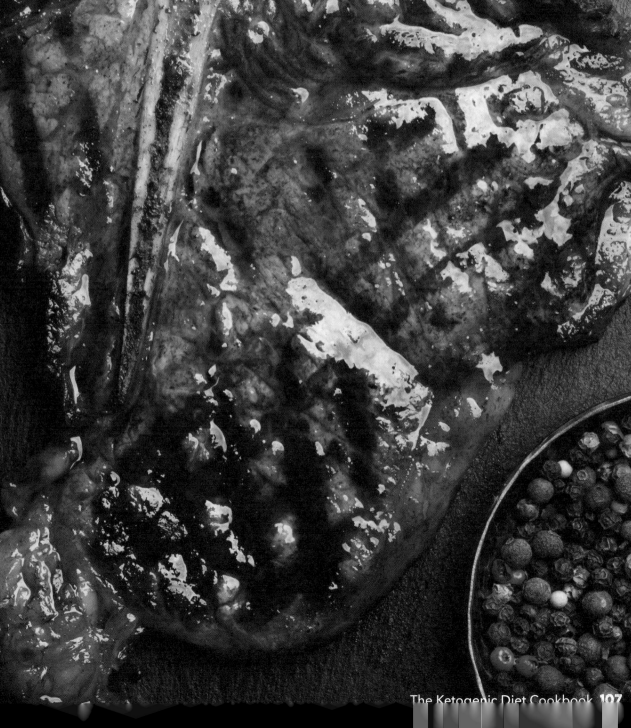

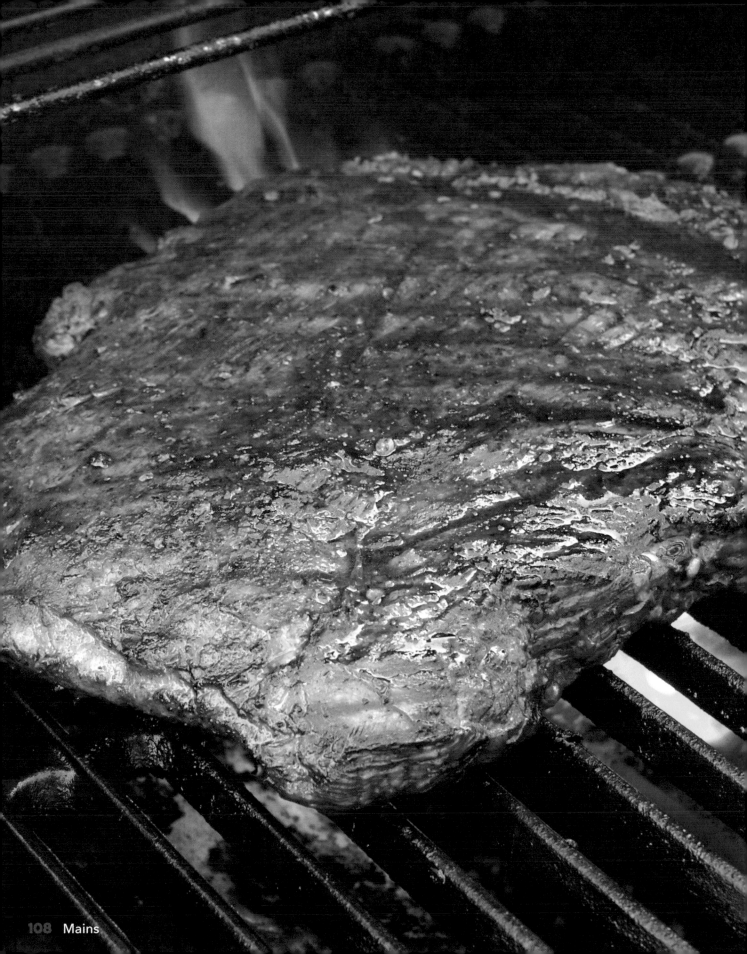

BASIC FLANK STEAK

SERVES: 2 / CALORIES: 584 / FAT: 44G / NET CARBS: 0G / PROTEIN: 48G

1 flank steak, about 1 to 1½ pounds

2 tablespoons extra-virgin olive oil

2 tablespoons butter

2 sprigs of rosemary, leaves removed

2 sprigs of thyme, leaves removes

Coarsely ground black pepper

Fresh sea salt

1. Remove the steak and rub with a mixture of the olive oil, rosemary, and thyme. Let rest at room temperature for 1 hour.

2. A half hour before cooking, prepare your gas or charcoal grill to medium-high heat.

3. When the grill is ready, about 400 to 450 degrees with the coals lightly covered with ash, season one side of the steak with half of the coarsely ground pepper and sea salt. Place the seasoned side of the steak on the grill and cook for about 4 to 5 minutes, seasoning the uncooked side of the steak while waiting. When the steak seems charred, gently flip and cook for 4 to 5 more minutes for medium-rare and 6 more minutes for medium. The steak should feel slightly firm if poked in the center.

4. Remove the steak from the grill and transfer to a large cutting board. Let stand for 6 to 8 minutes. Slice the steak diagonally into long, thin slices. Serve warm topped with the butter.

BIG TIP

Due to the flank's toughness, it is essential to slice this steak into very thin strips.

BISTECCA ALLA FIORENTINA

SERVES: 2 / CALORIES: 1052 / FAT: 61G / NET CARBS: 3G / PROTEIN: 118G

2 T-bone steaks, about ¾ to 1¼ inches thick (16 oz weight per steak)

4 cloves garlic, crushed

1 cup olive oil

1 sprig of rosemary, leaves removed

Coarsely ground black pepper

Fresh sea salt

1. Remove the steaks and place in a roasting pan or bowl. Then, rub the steaks with the rosemary, garlic, and ½ cup olive oil, and let rest at room temperature for 1 hour.

2. A half hour before cooking, prepare your gas or charcoal grill to medium-high heat.

3. When the grill is ready, about 400 to 450 degrees with the coals lightly covered with ash, season one side of the steak with half of the coarsely ground pepper and sea salt. Place the seasoned side of the steak on the grill and cook for 5 minutes, basting the unseasoned sides with the remaining olive oil every 30 seconds. Season the top sides with the remaining salt and pepper and then gently flip and cook for 4 to 6 more minutes, still basting until finished. The steak should feel slightly firm if poked in the center.

4. Remove the steaks from the grill and transfer to a large cutting board. Let stand for 6 to 8 minutes. Serve warm.

BIG TIP

The macros only include calories and fats for only 4 tbsp of the olive oil since you will not be consuming the entire cup and most of it will be using in cooking but not consumed by you. Same with the net carbs, if you do not eat the garlic it will be 0 net carbs.

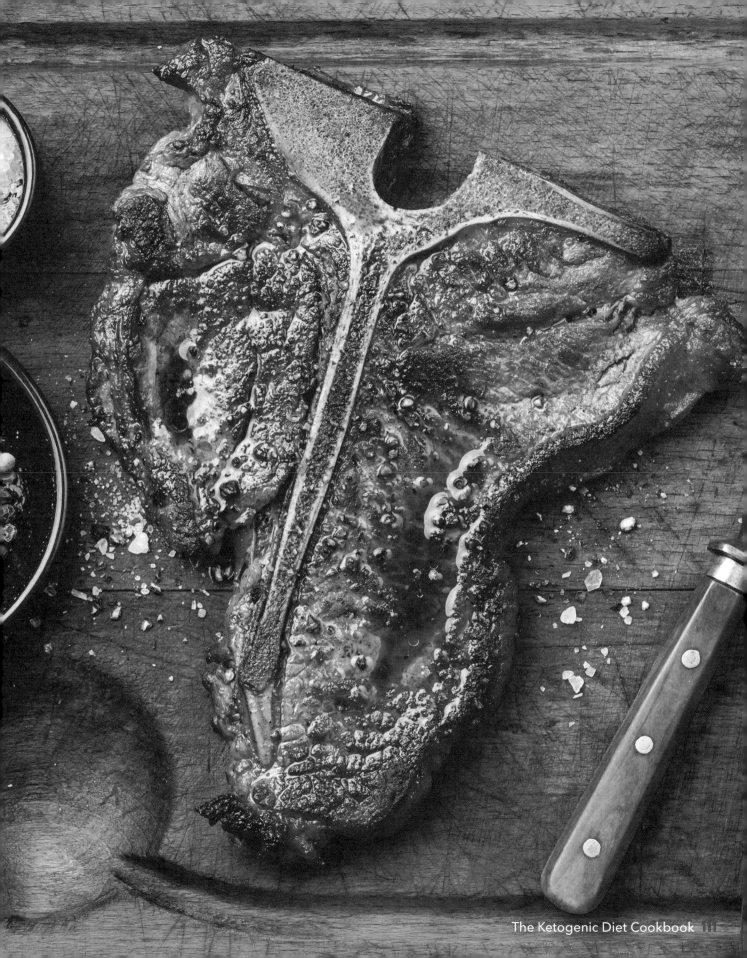

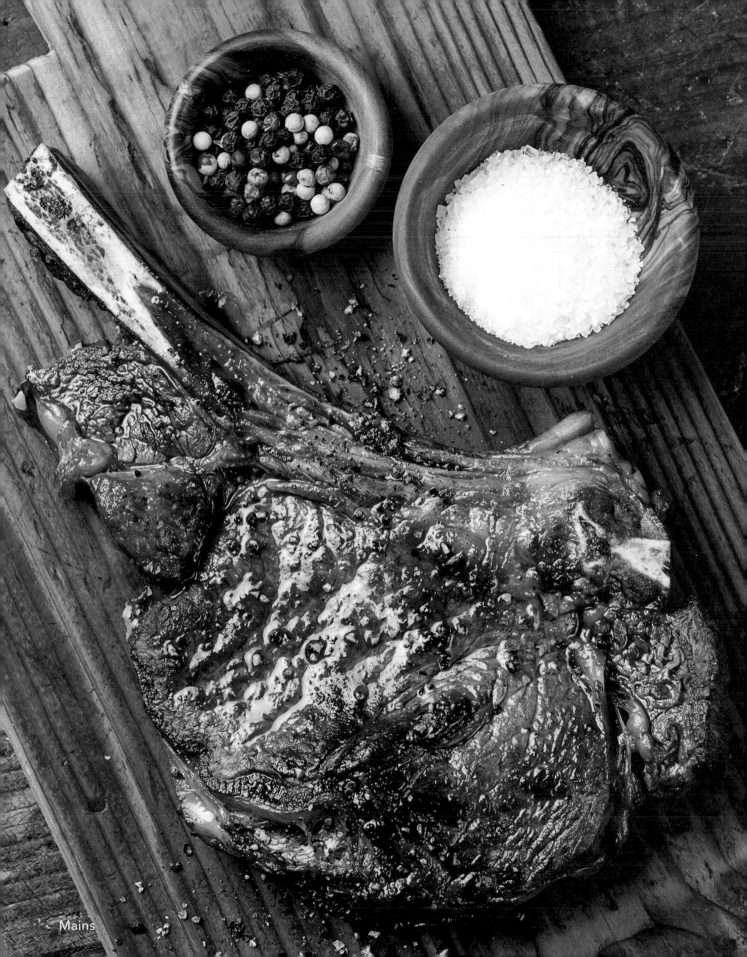

CHIPOTLE RIB EYE

SERVES: 2-3 / CALORIES: 909 / FAT: 69G / NET CARBS: 8G / PROTEIN: 60G

STEAK INGREDIENTS

2 bone-in rib eyes, about 1¼ to 1½ inches thick (16 oz weight per steak)

1 tablespoon extra-virgin olive oil

RUB INGREDIENTS

2 dry chipotle peppers, seeded and finely minced

1 tablespoon dried oregano

1 tablespoon dried cilantro

1 tablespoon coarsely ground black pepper

2 teaspoons ground cumin

1 teaspoon onion powder

½ teaspoon dry mustard

Fresh sea salt

1. Combine the rub ingredients and mix thoroughly.

2. Rub a very thin layer of olive oil to both sides of the steaks and then generously apply the dry rub, firmly pressing it all around the steak. Let rest at room temperature for at least 1 hour.

3. A half hour before cooking, prepare your gas or charcoal grill to medium-high heat.

4. When the grill is ready, at about 400 to 450 degrees with the coals lightly covered with ash, place the steaks on the grill and cook for about 6 to 7 minutes until blood begins to rise from the tops. When the steaks are charred, flip and cook for 4 to 5 more minutes for medium-rare and 5 to 6 more minutes for medium. The steaks should feel slightly firm if poked in the center.

5. Remove the steaks from the grill and transfer to a large cutting board. Let stand for 5 to 10 minutes, allowing the steaks to properly store their juices and flavor. Serve warm.

BIG TIP

To decrease the carbs replace the peppers with some cayenne pepper and for additional fat top the finished steak with butter.

CROWNED ROAST OF BEEF

SERVES: 12 / CALORIES: 966 / FAT: 83G / NET CARBS: 8G / PROTEIN: 87

A 10-rib rib roast (approx weight 10lbs)

3 tablespoons coarsely ground black pepper

3 tablespoons fresh sea salt

1 cup extra virgin olive oil

8 garlic cloves, minced

⅓ cup fresh thyme, coarsely chopped

⅓ cup fresh rosemary, coarsely chopped

4 tablespoons fresh sage, finely chopped

1. Remove the rib roast from the refrigerator and place it on cooling racks over a large carving board, bone-side down. To begin, you will need to french the rib roast. First, cut the meat that covers the bones. To do so, go about 2 inches down the ribs and using a sharp carving knife, cut through the meat until you reach the bone. Make a sharp cut and then cut up the bone so that the top of the meat can be peeled off.

2. Stand the rib roast up and starting with the left bone, cut down 1 to 2 inches along the bone, across to the next bone, and then back up so that you get a rectangular chunk of the meat to come apart from the space between the ribs. Do this to all the ribs, and then gently cut away the meat so that the ribs are left to stand openly and on their own. Using a paring knife, gently scrape away any bits of meat that still cling to the ribs.

3. Bring the meat together into a circle, cut about ½ to 1 inch into the meat side of the rib roast between each bone. Make your cuts even and leveled. Stand the rib roast and, pushing back the ends of the roast, form it into a tight crown. Note that because it's fairly difficult to crown a roast of beef, you may need to cut deeper than 1 inch between the ribs so that it allows for more flexibility. Using butcher's twine, tie the crown tightly so that it'll remain in that position while roasting—you'll need to tie the roast around the bones themselves, and also around the equator of the roast. Set aside.

4. Mix the coarsely ground black pepper and fresh sea salt in a small bowl. Using your hands, massage the seasoning into the rib roast.

5. In a small bowl whisk together the remaining ingredients. Using your hands, massage the paste into the rib roast. Let stand at room temperature for 30 minutes to 1 hour.

6. Preheat the oven to 450 degrees.

7. Place the standing rib roast in a large roasting pan on a large sheet of flat roasting racks. Cover the crown with aluminum foil so that it keeps the heat central. Roast at 450 degrees for 15 minutes so that the rib roast receives a nice initial searing. Lower the heat to 325 degrees and cook for another 2 to 3 hours, until the internal temperature of the meat reads 125 degrees for medium-rare. Baste the rib roast with its own juices every 30 minutes or so.

8. Remove the crown roast from the oven and place on a large serving piece. Let stand for 10 minutes before carving.

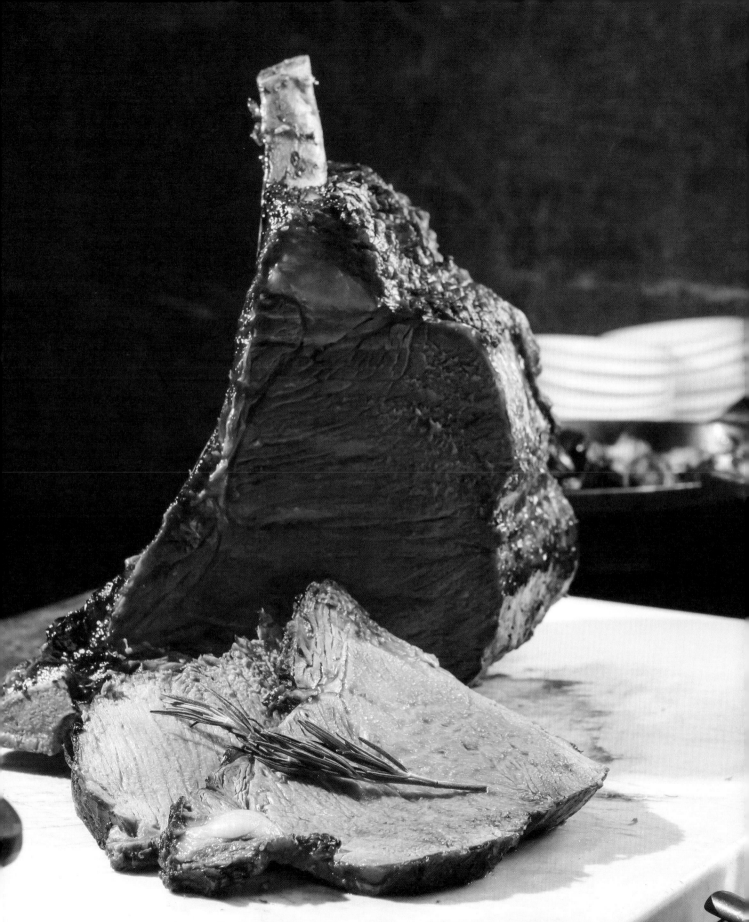

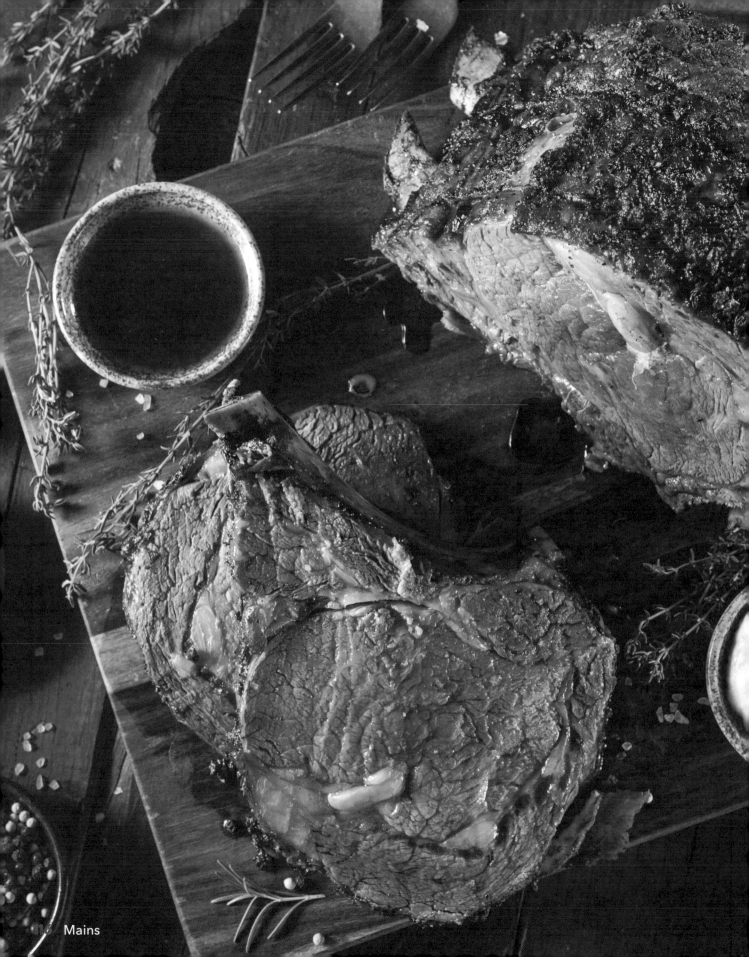

SLOW-COOKER PRIME RIB

SERVES: 4-8 / CALORIES: 686 / FAT: 47G / NET CARBS: 5G / PROTEIN: 53G

A 3- or 4-rib rib roast (4lbs in weight)

2 tablespoons coarsely ground black pepper

2 tablespoons fresh sea salt

4 garlic cloves, minced

1 teaspoon extra-virgin olive oil

4 sprigs fresh rosemary

4 sprigs fresh thyme

¼ cup dry red wine (preferably one you plan on serving at dinner)

1 cup chicken stock

1 bay leaf

1. Remove the rib roast from the refrigerator 1 hour before cooking. Using your hands, thoroughly apply the coarsely ground black pepper and fresh sea salt to the rib roast.

2. Next, in a small bowl, mix together the minced garlic and extra-virgin olive oil, and then apply to the roast. Let the roast stand at room temperature for about 1 hour.

3. Add the rosemary, thyme, red wine, chicken stock, and bay leaf to a slow cooker. Add the rib roast, fat side up, to the slow cooker. Turn the slow cooker to low and let cook for about 5 hours until, when tested with an instant-read thermometer, the internal temperature reads 130 degrees for medium-rare. Note that the marinade will not completely submerge the rib roast, so baste it or flip the meat halfway through the cooking time.

4. Remove the rib roast from the slow cooker and place on a large carving board. Let rest for 15 minutes before carving. As far as the leftover marinade goes, you can use this as the base of a sauce or gravy.

BIG TIP

The time to stand around and prepare a traditional full-course meal. With the slow cooker, a low temperature cooks the meat over a longer period of time, requiring little to no effort. Even here, when we consider the dry red wine and chicken stock that the prime rib cooks in for 5 hours, it's not entirely necessary to baste the roast every 30 minutes. Instead, just make sure that everything gets into the roast and that you cook it on the low setting. Other than that, just let the slow cooker do all the work for you.

PLENTIFUL PEPPERS AND BEEF IN LETTUCE WRAPS

SERVES: 10 / CALORIES: 261 / FAT: 16G / NET CARBS: 5G / PROTEIN: 22G

¼ cup extra-virgin olive oil

1 small onion, chopped

1 each of medium-sized yellow, red, and green bell peppers, cored, seeded and sliced

2 jalapeno peppers

1 teaspoon ancho chili powder

2 to 3 lbs sirloin beef, cut into thin strips

28 oz fresh tomatoes (pureed)

1 head crisp lettuce greens, like Romaine or endive, cut or broken into 3-inch sections

Grated cheddar or Pepperjack cheese for garnish

1. Heat the oil in a large skillet or saucepan. Add the onion and peppers and cook until just softening, about 5 minutes. Stir in the green chili peppers and ancho chili powder.

2. Transfer pepper mixture to the slow cooker. Top with the slices of steak, and pour the tomato puree over everything. Cover and cook on Low for 6 to 8 hours, or on High for 5 to 6 hours until the steak is tender.

3. To serve, put the steak and pepper mix in a bowl with a lid, and serve alongside a platter of prepared lettuce leaves. Fill the leaves as necessary so they don't get soggy and tear. Sprinkle grated cheese on top.

BIG TIP

If you want to wrap the peppers and beef in something besides lettuce leaves, consider low-carb tortillas. For extra tastiness, brush them on both sides with some olive oil and toast them on the grill for a minute or so a side. Macros do not include lettuce or grated cheese on top; log those as per the quantity you use.

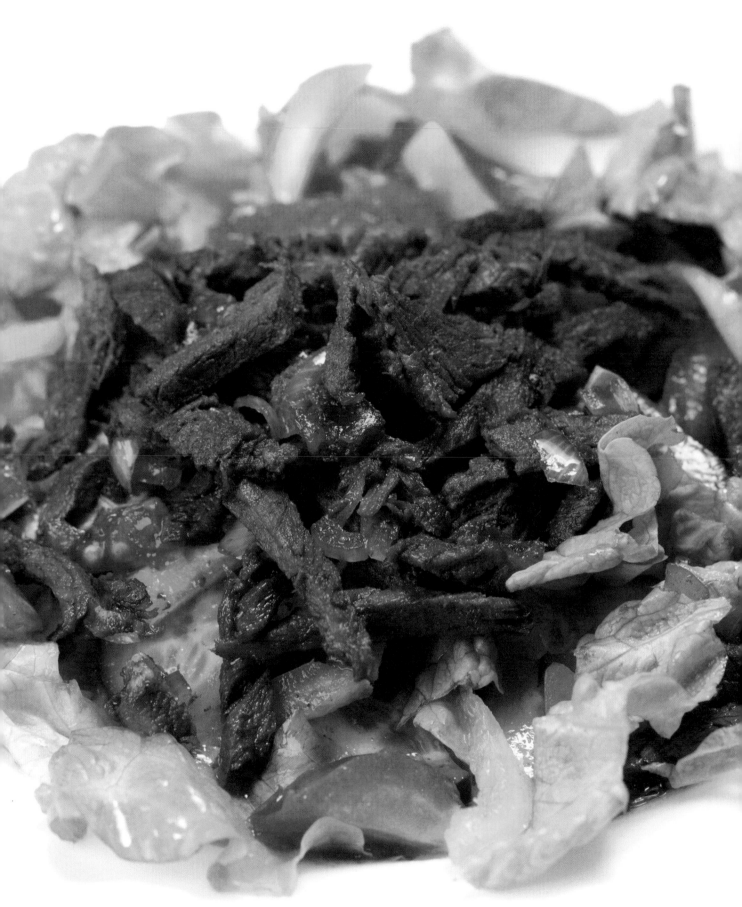

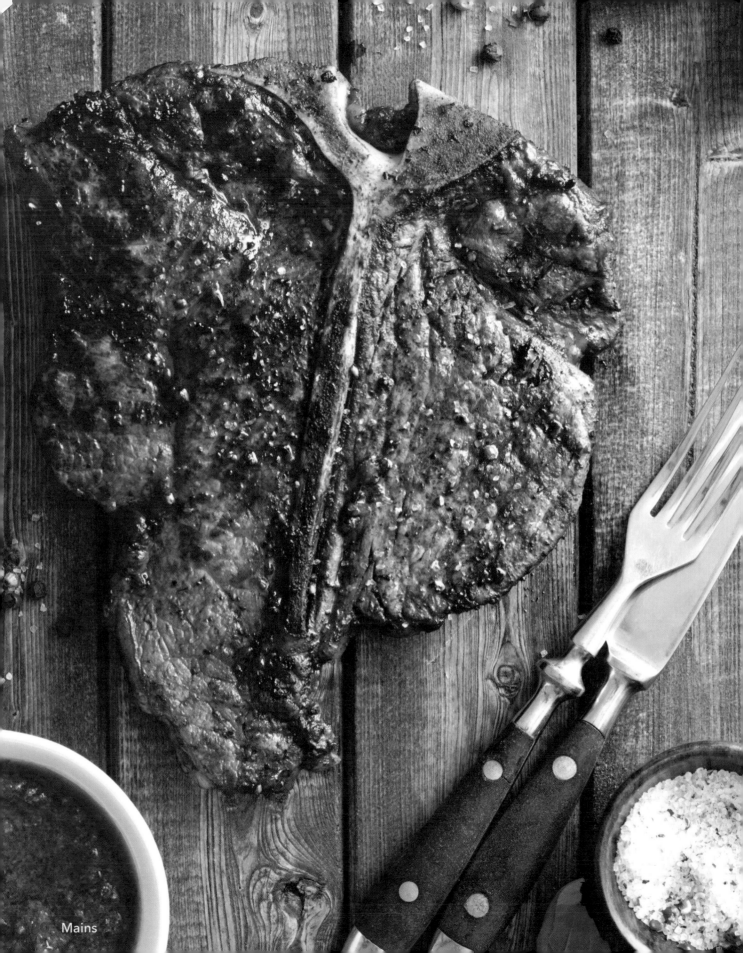

PORTERHOUSE WITH CHIMICHURRI SAUCE

STEAK SERVES: 4 / CALORIES: 479 / FAT: 39G / NET CARBS: 0G / PROTEIN: 30G
SAUCE CALORIES: 396 / FAT: 42G / NET CARBS: 4G / PROTEIN: 1G

STEAK INGREDIENTS

2 Porterhouse steaks, about 1½ inches thick (Approx 21 oz weight for both)

4 tablespoons extra-virgin olive oil

Coarsely ground black pepper

Fresh sea salt

SAUCE INGREDIENTS

½ cup red wine vinegar

4 garlic cloves, minced

1 shallot, minced

½ scallion, minced

1 Fresno chile, finely chopped (for additional spice, substitute for a minced habanero)

1 tablespoon fresh lemon juice

1 teaspoon fresh sea salt

½ cup flat-leaf parsley, minced

½ cup cilantro, minced

2 tablespoons, minced oregano

¾ cup extra-virgin olive oil

1. Rub both sides of the steaks with olive oil and let rest at room temperature for about 1 hour.

2. A half hour before cooking, prepare your gas or charcoal grill to medium-high heat.

3. While you wait, combine the vinegar, garlic, shallot, scallion, Fresno chile, lemon juice, and salt in a medium bowl and let rest for 15 minutes. Next, add the parsley, cilantro, and oregano, then gradually whisk in the olive oil. Set aside.

4. When the grill is ready, at about 400 to 450 degrees with the coals lightly covered with ash, season one side of the steaks with half of the coarsely ground pepper and sea salt, as well as a very light brush of the sauce along the bone.

5. Place the seasoned-sides of the steaks on the grill and cook for about 5 to 6 minutes, seasoning the tops of the steaks while waiting. Again, lightly trace the bone with the sauce. When the steaks are charred, flip and cook for 4 to 5 more minutes for medium-rare, and 6 to 7 for medium. The steaks should feel slightly firm if poked in the center.

6. Remove the steaks from the grill and transfer to a large cutting board. Let stand for 10 minutes, allowing the steaks to properly store their juices and flavor. Serve warm with the Chimichurri sauce on the side.

BIG TIP

The Argentinian Chimichurri sauce goes well with any steak. It can be used as marinade, though this is sometimes a little risky because of the light kick from the Fresno chile. I suggest serving the chimichurri sauce on the side, and for those who would like even more heat in the sauce, substitute a habanero in place for the Fresno chile!

POT ROAST WITH MUSHROOM IN TRUFFLE OIL

SERVES: 8 / CALORIES: 405 / FAT: 23G / NET CARBS: 3G / PROTEIN: 46G

4 lbs chuck roast

4 tablespoons herb-infused extra-virgin olive oil

4 tablespoons butter

2 cloves garlic, minced

1 lb fresh white mushrooms, sliced

½ lb "babybellas"—small Portobello mushrooms, stems removed

2 cups beef broth

Salt and pepper

½ cup sour cream

1. Place roast in the slow cooker.

2. Heat oil and butter in a skillet over medium heat. Add garlic and both types of fresh mushrooms. Stir and cook until mushrooms soften, about 5 minutes. Remove from heat.

3. Transfer the mushroom mixture to the slow cooker. Top with the beef broth. Cover and cook on Low for 8 to 10 hours or on High for 6 to 8 hours. Season with salt and pepper.

4. Stir in sour cream just before serving.

─ BIG TIP ─

Cooking the mushrooms in an herb-infused olive oil can bring out their earthiness even more. Try popular types like basil/garlic, or pepper/garlic. If you don't have any handy, just go with extra virgin olive oil and add a teaspoon of sage after cooking the mushrooms.

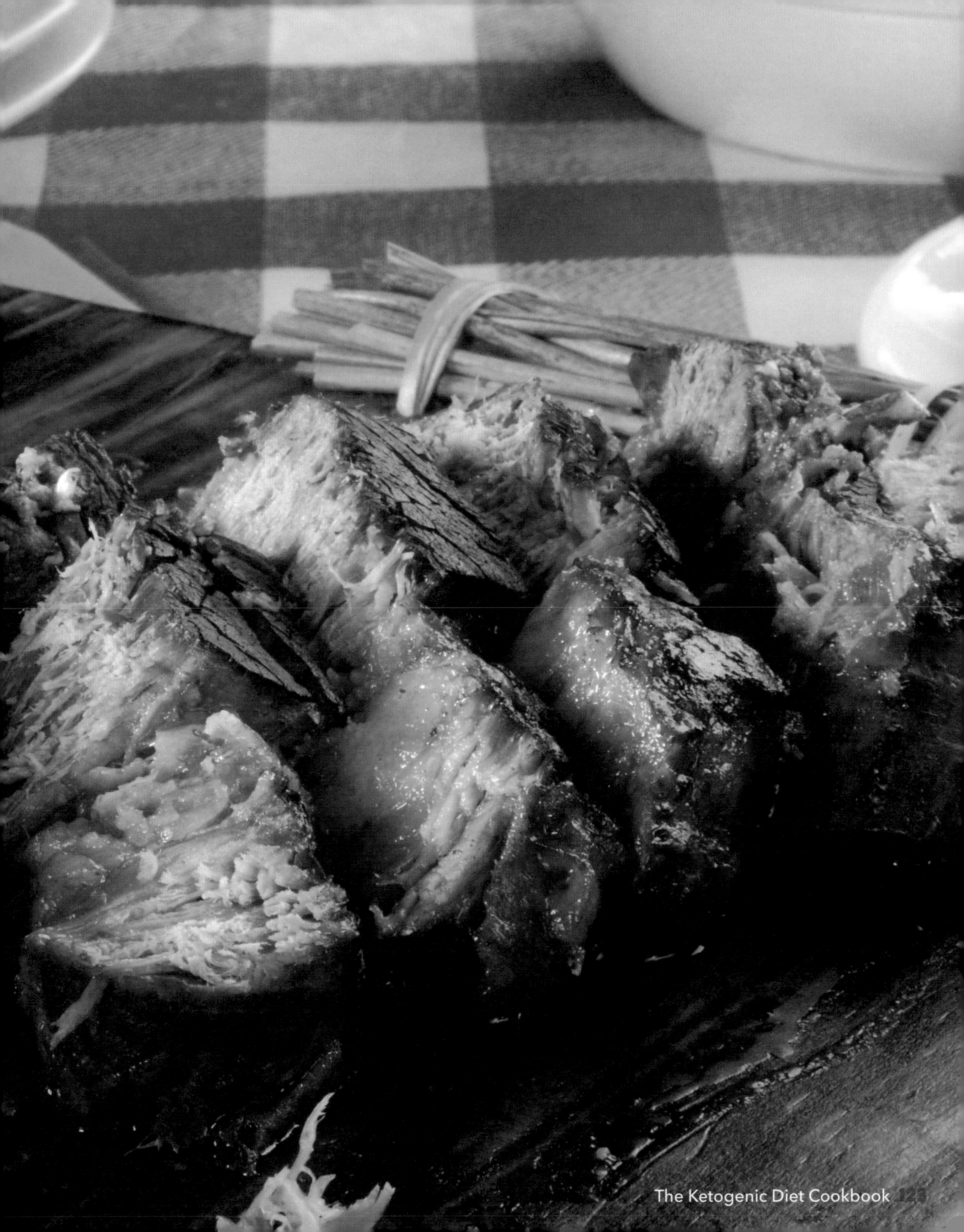

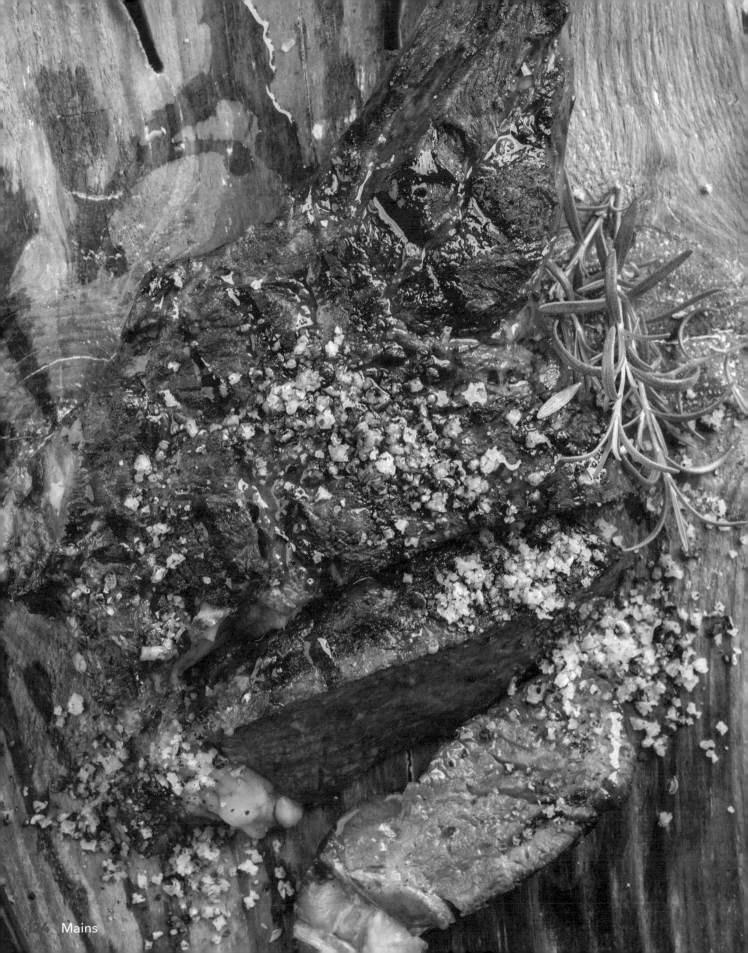

Mains

B&B PRIME RIB DINNER

SERVES: 8 / CALORIES: 736 / FAT: 64G / NET CARBS: 0G / PROTEIN: 77G

A 6-rib rib roast (6lbs weight)

3 tablespoons fresh sea salt

3 tablespoons coarsely ground black pepper

¼ cup extra-virgin olive oil

1. In a small bowl, combine the fresh sea salt and coarsely ground black pepper and mix thoroughly. Using your hands, pat the seasoning firmly onto the rib roast and then brush with the extra-virgin olive oil. Let stand at room temperature for 1 hour before cooking.

2. Set a large plancha skillet across two burners on the stovetop and set to high heat. (You may also use a cast-iron skillet large enough to fit the rib roast.) Place the rib roast fatty side down on the plancha skillet and sear for 15 minutes, until a crust is formed. When crusted, remove from the skillet and place on cooling racks set over a large carving board. Let rest for 15 minutes.

3. Preheat the oven to 325 degrees.

4. Place the rib roast meat side up on a rack in a roasting pan and transfer to the oven. Roast for 2 to 3 hours, basting every 30 minutes or so with its own juices, until its internal temperature reads 125 degrees for medium-rare.

5. Remove the rib roast from the oven and let rest for 10 minutes before carving, allowing it to properly store its juices and flavor.

SKIRT STEAK WITH OLIVE TAPENADE

SERVES: 4 / CALORIES: 1000 / FAT: 66G / NET CARBS: 5G / PROTEIN: 1G

STEAK INGREDIENTS

2 skirt steaks, (1 lbs each)

2 tablespoons extra-virgin olive oil

Coarsely ground black pepper

Fresh sea salt

TAPENADE INGREDIENTS

1 cup Niçoise olives, pitted and chopped

½ cup olive oil

½ small shallot, minced

1 garlic clove, minced

1 sprig of rosemary, leaves removed and finely minced

1 anchovy fillet (optional)

1 tablespoon basil, finely chopped

1 tablespoon flat-leaf parsley, finely chopped

1 tablespoon capers, minced

1 tablespoon thyme

1 teaspoon red pepper flakes

1. Rub both sides of the steaks with olive oil and let rest at room temperature for about 1 hour.

2. While waiting, combine the tapenade ingredients in a medium bowl and mix thoroughly. Set aside.

3. A half hour before cooking, prepare your gas or charcoal grill to extremely high heat.

4. When the grill is ready, about 500 to 600 degrees with the coals lightly covered with ash, season the steaks with the coarsely ground pepper and sea salt. Place the steaks on the grill and spoon the tapenade onto the top of each steak. Cook for about 3 minutes and then flip. Again, add the tapenade and cook for about 2 to 3 minutes for medium-rare, and 3 to 4 for medium. The steaks should be very charred and slightly firm if poked in the center.

5. Remove the steaks from the grill and transfer to a large cutting board. Let stand for 5 to 10 minutes. Slice the steak diagonally into long, thin slices and arrange the tapenade on the side. Serve warm. The tri-tip should be slightly firm and if an instant-read thermometer is inserted into the roast's thickest section, it should read around 125 degrees.

BIG TIP

The skirt steak is often referred to as the chewiest piece of meat. However, because of how thin it is, it is very easy to overcook the steak, which then promotes the chewiness. As such, grill these steaks over direct heat and make sure not to cook past medium.

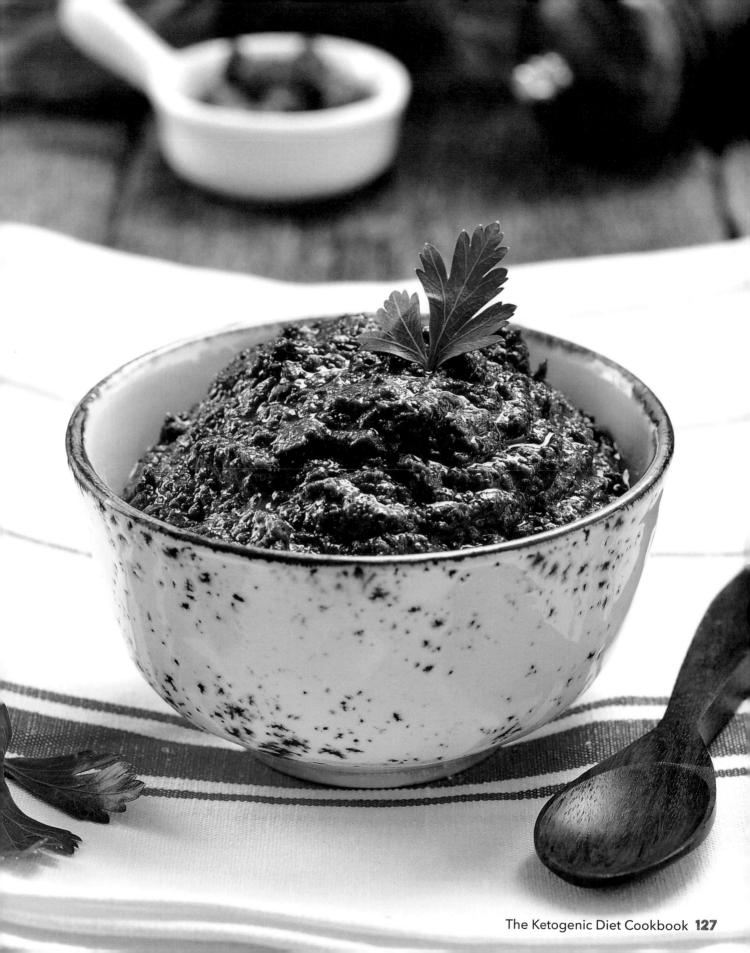

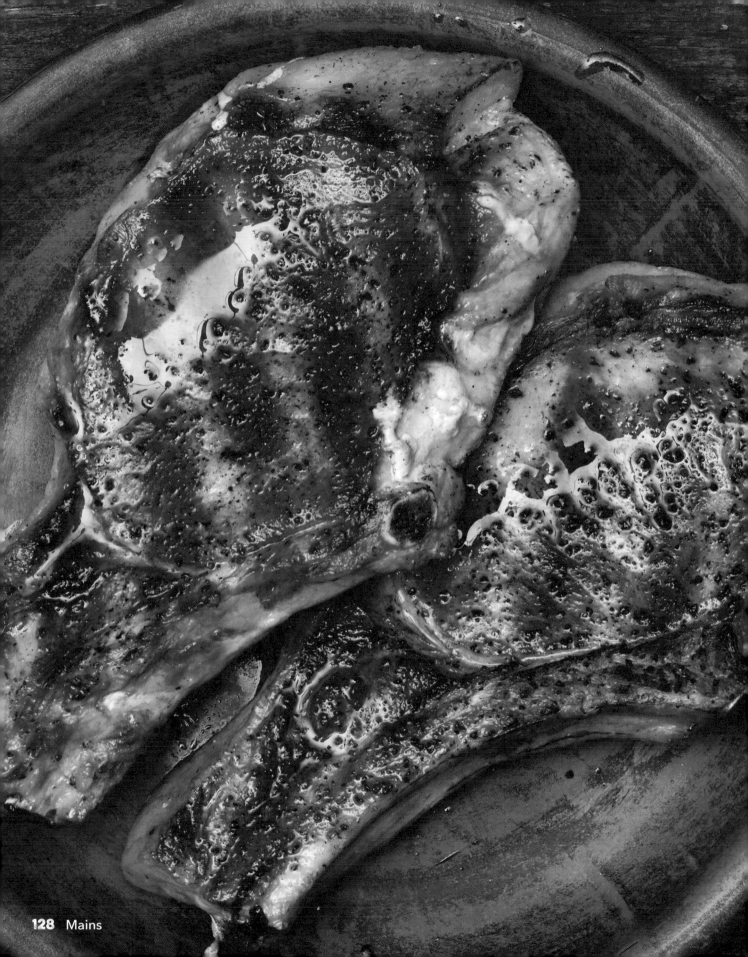

PALEO PORK CHOPS

SERVES: 4 / CALORIES: 295 / FAT: 21G / NET CARBS: 1G / PROTEIN: 24G

2 cloves garlic, minced

1 cup fresh basil leaves, minced

2 tablespoons lemon juice

2 tablespoons extra-virgin olive oil

1 pinch salt and pepper

4 pork loin chops, bone-in

1. In a small bowl, combine the garlic, basil, lemon juice, extra-virgin olive oil, salt and pepper. Spread over the pork chops and marinate for 30–45 minutes.

2. Grill over medium heat for about 4 minutes on each side, or until the pork chops are tender.

BIG TIP

The trick to cooking pork chops isn't in the seasoning: Everything hinges on how long you cook the meat. Pork chops tend to dry out very suddenly—if you have a meat thermometer on hand, check the internal temperature regularly until it reads 145 degrees F, then remove from heat immediately.

EVERYDAY TURKEY BREAST

SERVES: 6 / CALORIES: 512 / FAT: 15G / NET CARBS: 0G / PROTEIN: 91G

4-lb boneless, skinless turkey breast

½ teaspoon salt

¼ teaspoon pepper

1 tablespoon fresh rosemary, chopped

1 tablespoon fresh parsley, chopped

½ cup chicken stock or broth

6 tablespoons melted butter

1. Place the turkey in the slow cooker. Sprinkle with salt and pepper, add herbs, and add stock.

2. Cover and cook on Low for 7 to 9 hours or on High for 4 to 6 hours, or until the meat is cooked through.

3. Pour melted butter over before serving.

BIG TIP

You might find yourself preparing this at the end of every week so you can slice into it as your week gets busy. It makes a lovely, finished meat that can be used to top salads, roll in lettuce leaves, or even eat out of the fridge.

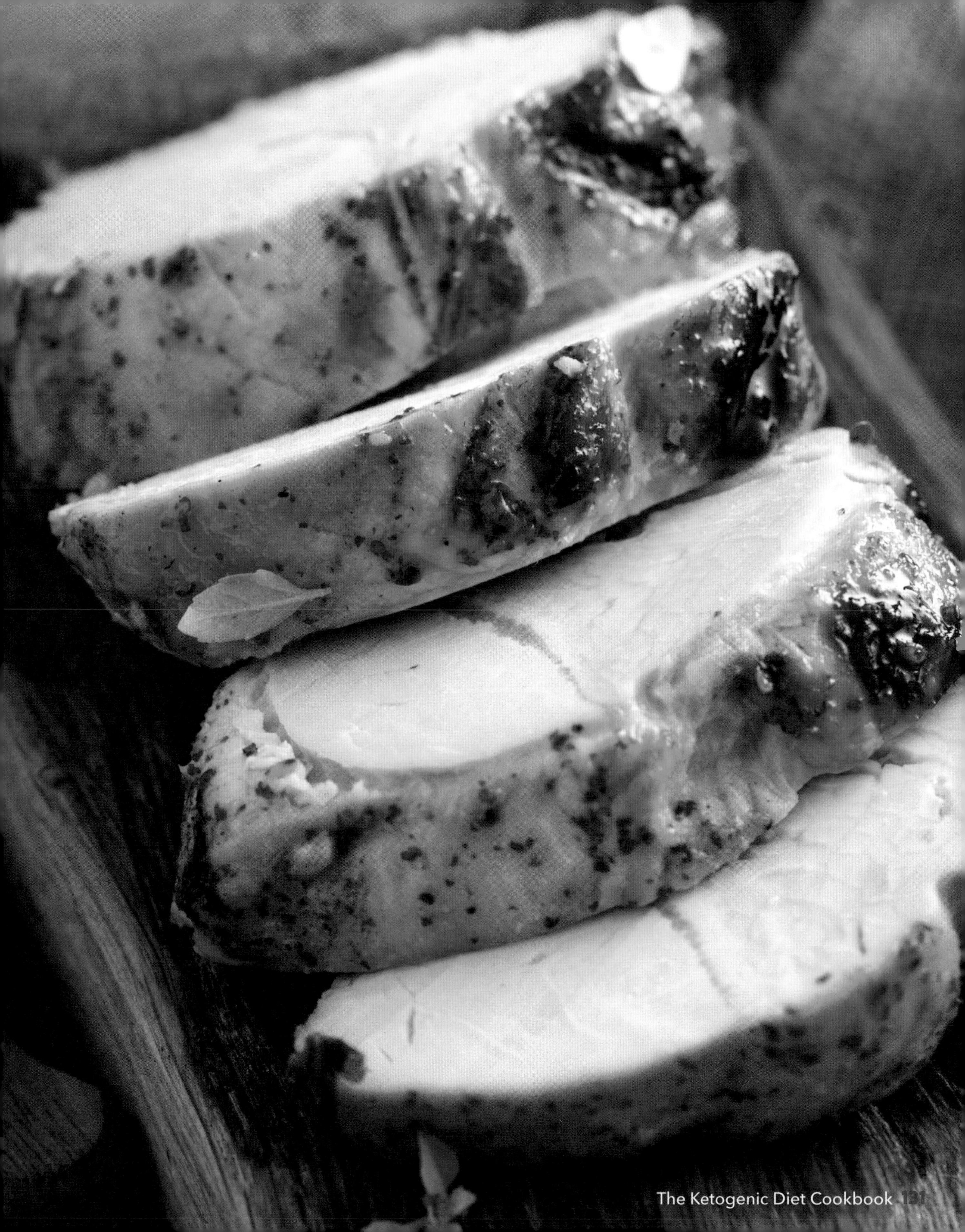

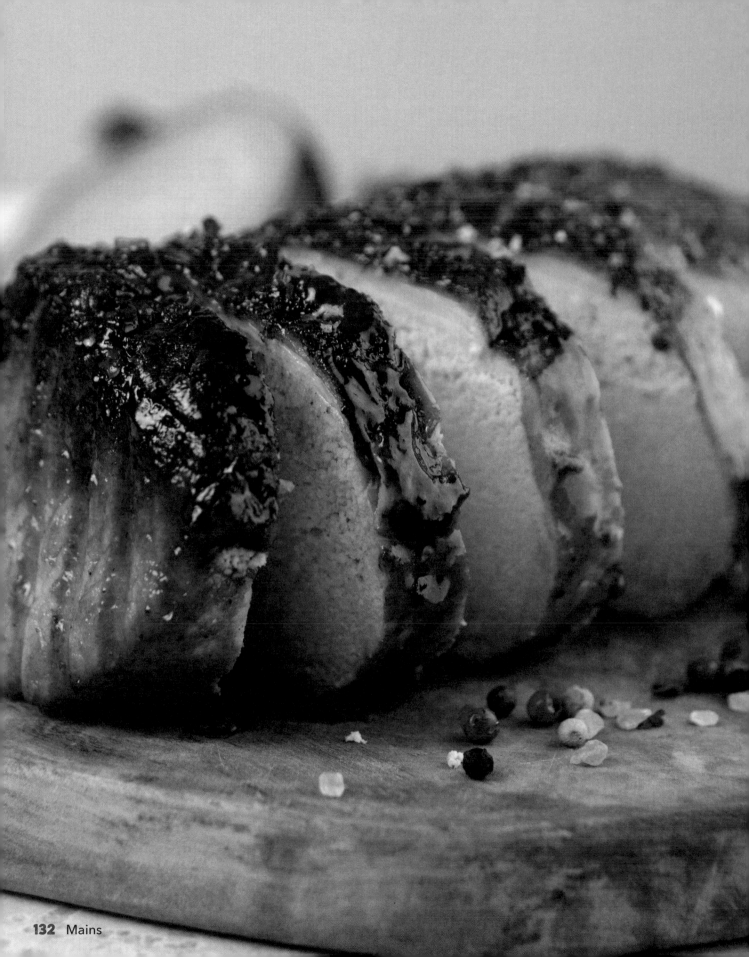

BASIC GRILLED ROAST PORK LOIN

SERVES: 5-6 / CALORIES: 365 / FAT: 21G / NET CARBS: 0G / PROTEIN: 43G

---

5 tablespoons of extra-virgin olive oil

1 or 2 sprigs of fresh rosemary

2¼ pounds loin of pork

Fresh sea salt

Coarsely ground black pepper

1. Fire up your grill and allow the coals to settle into a temperature of about 350 degrees. While the grill is heating, slowly sauté the olive oil and rosemary in a cast-iron or All-Clad–style high heat–friendly pan. Be sure the pan is oven-and-grill friendly, as you will be placing this pan directly onto your grill.

2. After the oil and rosemary have been thoroughly heated and the flavors of the sprigs are infused throughout the oil (about 10 to 12 minutes), rub your pork loin with sea salt and fresh cracked pepper to your desired seasoning, and place the pork loin into the pan, turning it so the entire loin is covered with the heated oil.

3. Baste for 5 to 10 minutes at a medium heat until the loin begins to brown. Once your grill has reached the desired temperature, move the entire pan to your grill grate.

4. Cover your grill and allow the pork to cook for 45 minutes, turning and basting the pork occasionally so all sides are thoroughly browned from the heat of the hot pan.

5. At about 45 minutes, remove the pork loin from the pan and place directly on the grate. Continue to baste your pork loin using the infused oil from the pan, turning the loin evenly so the entire roast is meets the heat side of your grill. Baste and turn for an additional 15 or so minutes or until the roast meets your desired temperature.

6. Remove from fire and let the loin rest for 10 to 12 minutes. Carve and serve with sides of your choice.

BIG TIP

For any oven-to-grill recipe, avoid using any cookware that has a plastic, wood, or synthetic-type handle. It is best if the pan has rounded sides, high enough to prevent the oil from spilling or flaring up when basting. Top each serving with a tablespoon of butter to add fat macros to the dish.

BRAISED AND GRILLED PORK WITH ROSEMARY

SERVES: 6 / CALORIES: 505 / FAT: 39G / NET CARBS: 3G / PROTEIN: 42G

2 sprigs of rosemary (remove needles from their stems)

2¼ pounds of boneless pork loin

8 tablespoons of extra-virgin olive oil

1 garlic clove, crushed

½ onion, chopped

¾ cup white wine

1 tablespoon white vinegar

Fresh sea salt

Coarsely ground black pepper

1. To enhance the flavor and to prevent the rosemary from searing completely off during the cooking process, push the rosemary needles into the meat. This will help infuse the flavor throughout the pork. Leave a little bit of each rosemary sprig sticking out to catch and burn from the flame; this adds to the flavor.

2. Brush and coat the roast with olive oil.

3. Place the roast into a deep sauté pan that can withstand the direct heat of your grill. Place the remaining oil into the pan, turning and cooking the pork evenly on all sides until it reaches a lovely golden brown.

4. Add the garlic, onion, and remaining rosemary, and let the meat and seasoning cook together for about an hour. If you can control the temperature of your grill, bring the heat down so everything may simmer together for 1½ hours.

5. Just before the pork appears to be done, remove it from the pan and place it directly on the grill to sear off the rosemary sprigs and to gracefully char the exterior to your preference.

6. Remove the roast from the grill, and let it stand for 10 to 12 minutes. Slice thin before serving, and use some of the cooked juices as a light gravy if the pork happens to get slightly overdone.

BIG TIP

For summer flavors, consider substituting 2 sprigs of rosemary with 3 tablespoons freshly chopped dill.

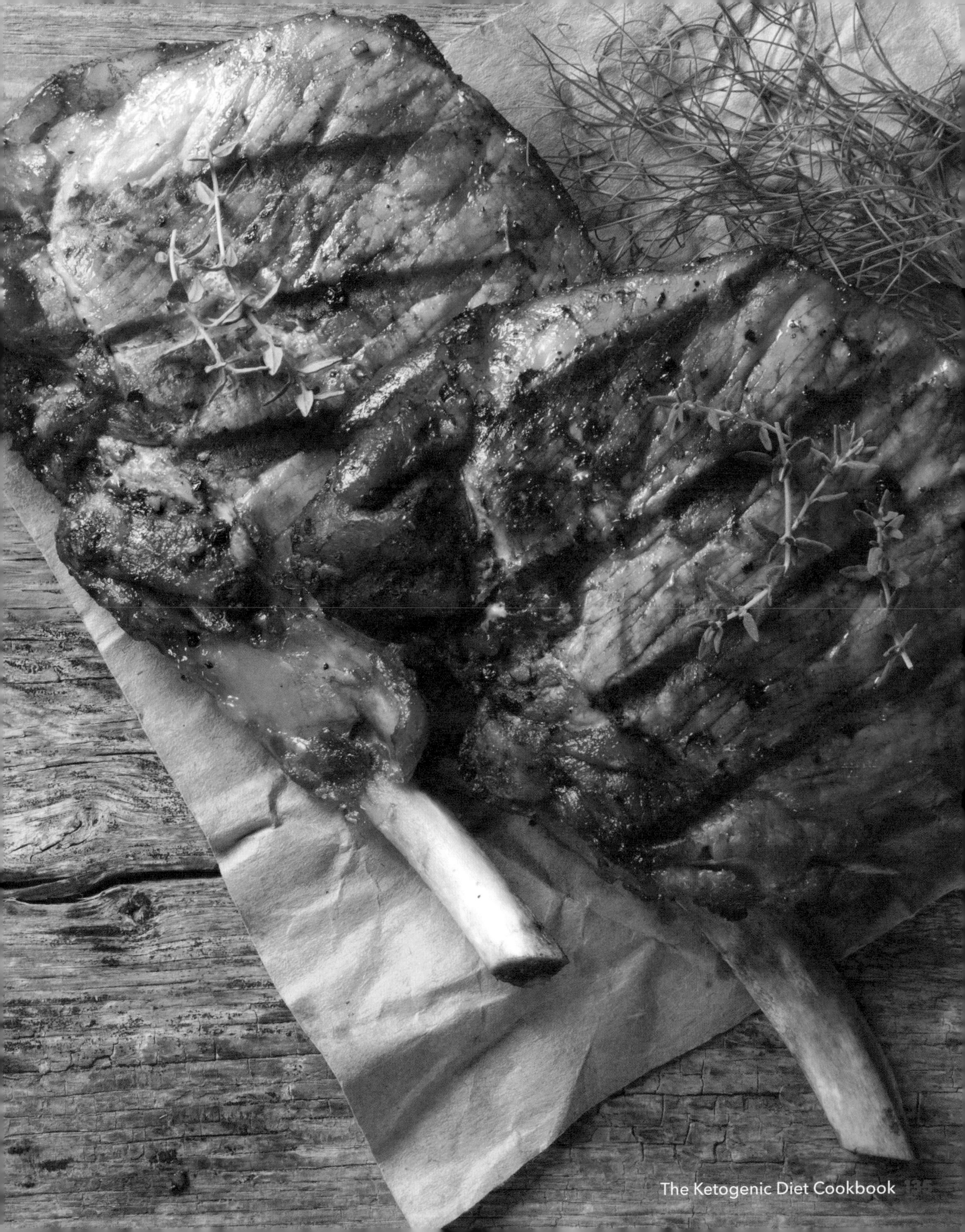

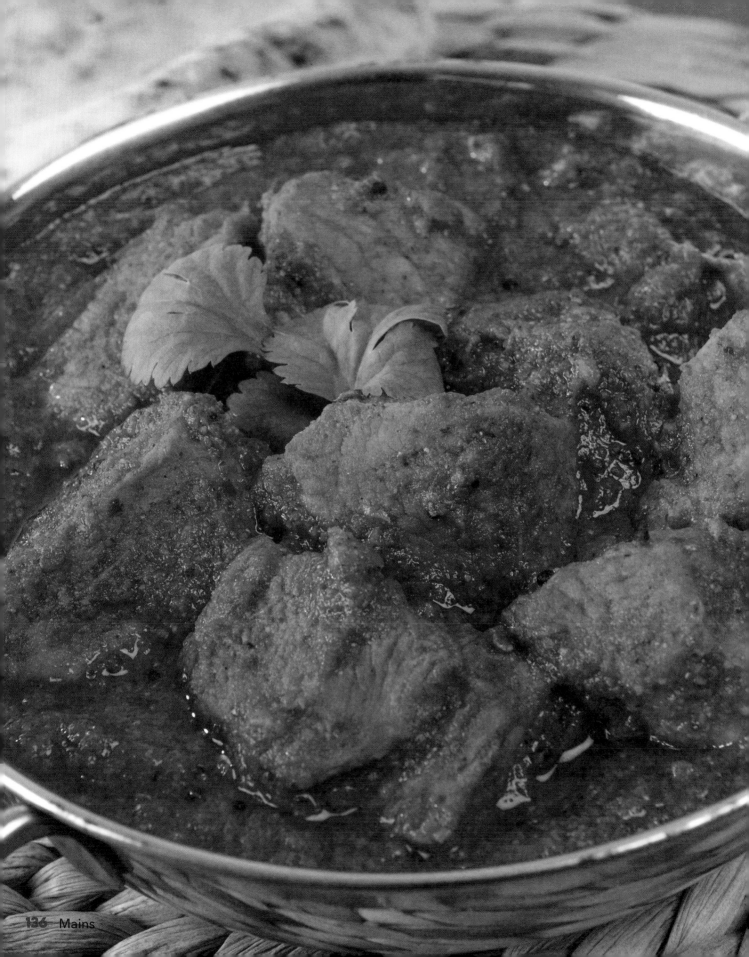

PORK VINDALOO

SERVES: 6/ CALORIES: 590 / FAT: 41G / NET CARBS: 7G / PROTEIN: 46G

2 tablespoons extra-virgin olive oil

1 large onion, sliced thin

6 chilies, such as jalapenos, habaneros, or a combination, seeded and sliced (wear gloves to do this)

1 teaspoon turmeric

1 teaspoon ground coriander

1½ teaspoons garam masala

½ teaspoon cinnamon

2½ lbs pork butt, trimmed and cut into cubes

2 tablespoons apple cider vinegar

2 tablespoons fresh ginger, grated

10 cloves garlic, peeled

1 teaspoon dry mustard powder

16 oz fresh tomatoes chopped finely

2 cups water

1. Heat oil in a skillet over medium-high heat and add slices of 2 onions. Cook, stirring frequently, for about 3 minutes, until onions are translucent.

2. Add tomatoes, chilies, turmeric, coriander, garam masala, and cinnamon, stirring constantly to coat the onions, tomatoes and chilies with the spices. Remove from heat.

3. Put pork chunks into the slow cooker, and add the onion, tomato spice mix. Add the garlic cloves, cider vinegar, ginger, dry mustard and stir well. Add water over the pork mixture. Cover and cook on Low for 6 to 8 hours or on High for 4 to 5 hours.

BIG TIP

The whole cloves of garlic in this recipe are a treat to eat. The garlic gets soft and loses its bite and is instead infused with the other spices.

SPICY SPARERIBS

SERVES: 6 / CALORIES: 402 / FAT: 34G / NET CARBS: 1G / PROTEIN: 20G

2 tablespoons extra-virgin olive oil

3 lbs country-style spareribs (thick cut)

1 teaspoon cayenne pepper

Salt and freshly ground pepper

8 oz fresh tomatoes (pureed)

1 teaspoon cumin

½ teaspoon cinnamon

½ teaspoon ancho chili powder

½ teaspoon garlic powder

1. Put the olive oil in a baking dish. Put the ribs in the dish and stir and toss them to coat with olive oil. Sprinkle the oiled ribs with cayenne, salt, and pepper. Place in the slow cooker.

2. In a bowl, combine the tomatoes, water, cumin, cinnamon, ancho chili powder, and garlic powder. Stir. Pour over ribs. Cover and cook on Low for 8 to 10 hours.

3. Skim fat off the top, finish the ribs on the grill if you want them crunchy on the outside, and serve the sauce on the side.

BIG TIP

As you make the spicy sauce with the tomatoes, taste it and consider varying the flavor by using more or less of the listed spices, and even adding something else you like. If you want something a bit less smoky, substitute red pepper flakes for the ancho chili powder. A word of caution, though: Don't overdo the cinnamon.

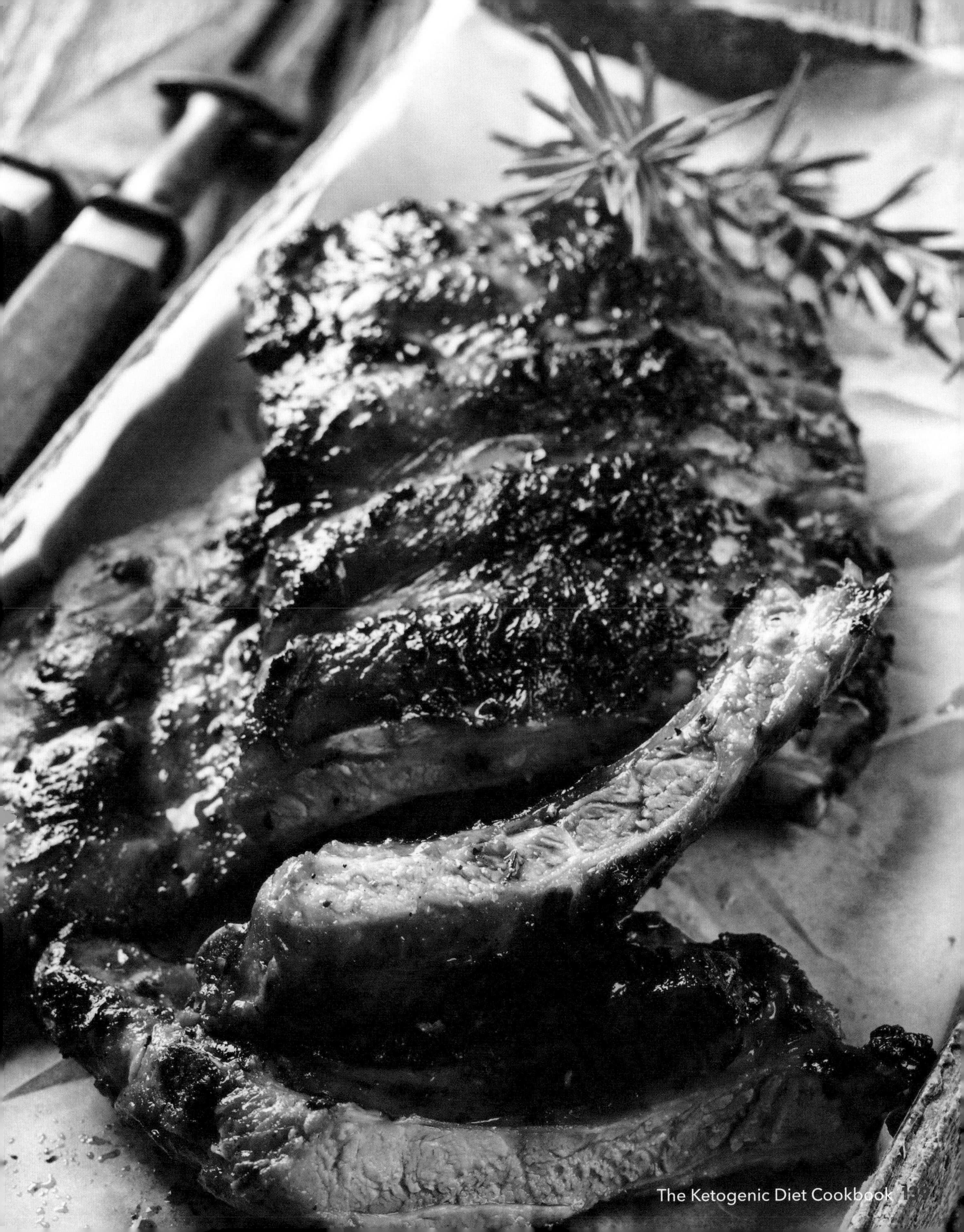

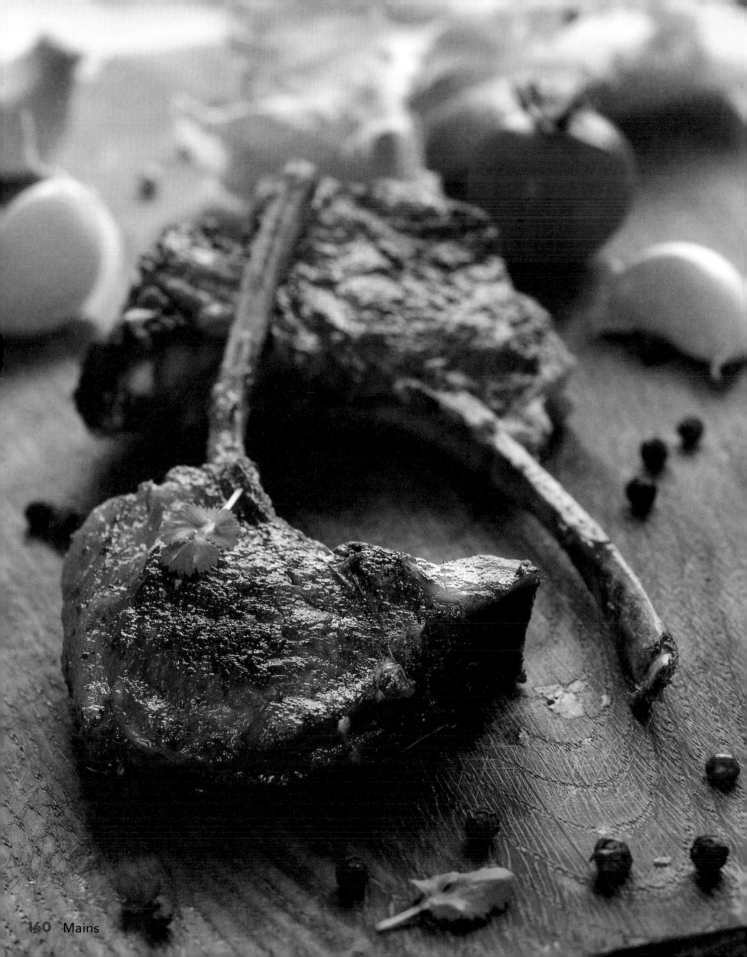

LAMB CHOPS WITH ROSEMARY AND LEMON

SERVES: 4 / CALORIES: 356 / FAT: 22G / NET CARBS: 3G / PROTEIN: 33G

4 tablespoons fresh-squeezed lemon juice (no seeds)

2 tablespoons fresh rosemary leaves, chopped

2 cloves garlic, pressed

Salt and pepper to taste

8 lamb chops (Approx weight 24oz with bone in)

1. Preheat the broiler on high. Position a rack to be about 5 to 7 inches away from the heat. Put the skillet in the oven so it gets hot.

2. In a bowl, combine the lemon juice and rosemary. Press the garlic into the mix and season with salt and pepper. Using your hands, rub the chops in the mix, being sure to coat both sides and distribute evenly. Put the chops on a platter.

3. When the skillet is hot, take it out and position the chops in it so they fit. Return to the rack under the broiler and cook for about 5 minutes. Since the skillet is already hot, the lamb is cooking on both sides at once.

4. Remove from the oven, let rest for a minute, and serve.

BIG TIP

Lamb chops are an indulgence, for sure, so if you're going to splurge, be sure to follow this recipe when preparing them. The rosemary, garlic, and lemon seasoning bring out the earthy goodness of the chops to perfection.

LAMB CHOPS WITH PAPRIKA-SALT RUB

SERVES: 4 / CALORIES: 706 / FAT: 51G / NET CARBS: 0G / PROTEIN: 48G

12 lamb rib chops, each about 1 inch thick (approx weight 36 oz)

2 tablespoons extra-virgin olive oil

2 tablespoons smoked paprika

1 tablespoon cumin seeds

2 teaspoons coriander seeds

½ teaspoon cayenne pepper

Coarsely ground black pepper

Fresh sea salt

1. An hour before grilling, brush the meat on the lamb rib chops with olive oil and let stand at room temperature.

2. In a small bowl, mix together the remaining ingredients to make the paprika-salt rub. Using your hands, generously apply the rub to the lamb rib chops.

3. Prepare your gas or charcoal grill to medium-high heat.

4. When the grill is ready, at about 400 to 450 degrees with the coals lightly covered with ash, place the lamb rib chops on the grill and cook for about 4 minutes or until the spices have browned. Turn the chops and cook for another 3 to 4 minutes for medium-rare, 4 to 5 minutes for medium.

5. Transfer the lamb rib chops to a large carving board and let stand for 5 minutes before serving.

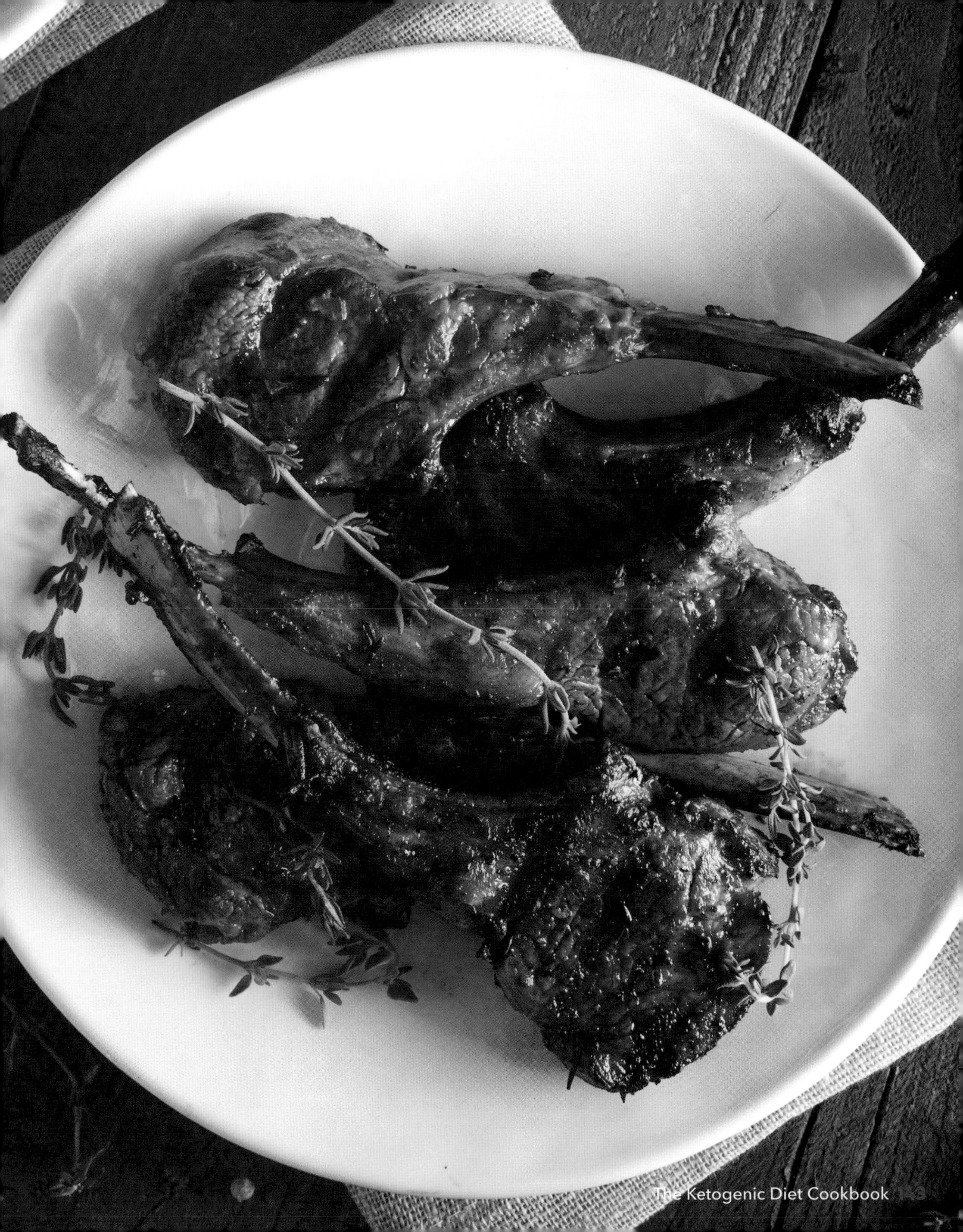

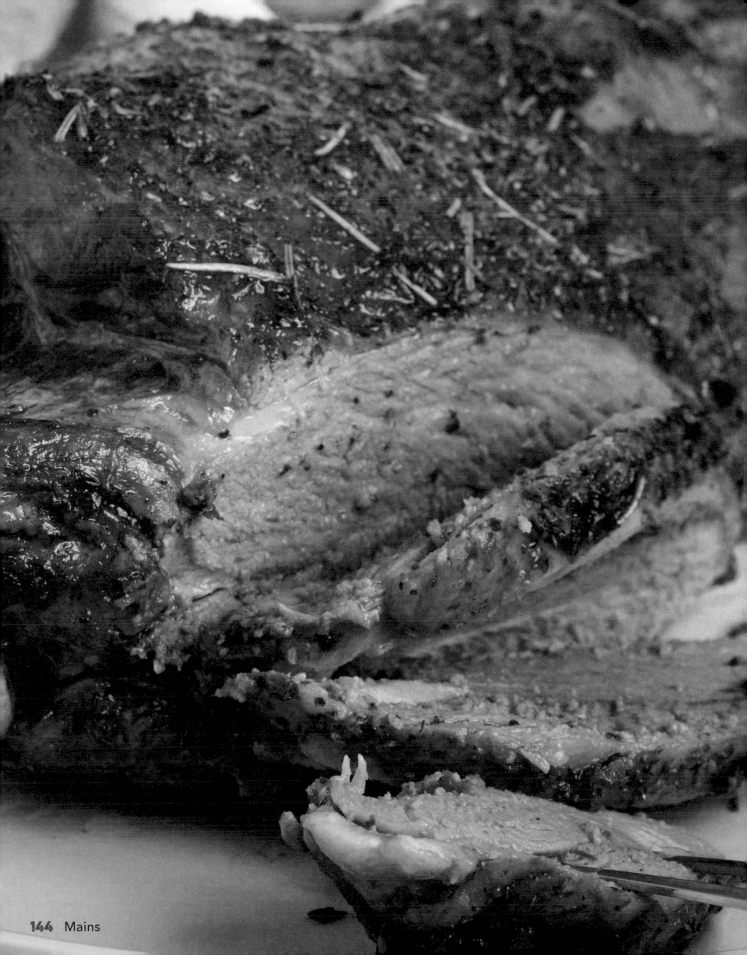

LAZY LADY'S LEG OF LAMB

SERVES: 8 / CALORIES: 505 / FAT: 34G / NET CARBS: 1G / PROTEIN: 48G

1 bone-in leg of lamb (shank removed)

1 tablespoon extra-virgin olive oil

½ teaspoon sea salt

½ teaspoon freshly ground black pepper

1 teaspoon fresh rosemary, chopped

1 teaspoon fresh mint, chopped

3 cloves garlic, minced

1. Put the extra-virgin olive oil in your hands and rub the oil all over the lamb.

2. Put the lamb in the slow cooker and sprinkle it all over with the salt, pepper, rosemary, mint, and garlic, rubbing the spices onto the meat.

3. Cover and cook on Low for 6 to 8 hours. Do not cook on High.

4. Season with additional salt and pepper if desired.

BIG TIP

Serve the lamb with a lively sugar-free mint sauce. Make it by chopping together ½ cup fresh mint leaves and ½ cup fresh parsley leaves. Stir in about ½ cup olive oil, salt and pepper to taste, and a squeeze or so of fresh lemon juice. If you feel it needs some sweetening, stir in a teaspoon of honey.

MARINATED LAMB KEBABS WITH MINT CHIMICHURRI

SERVES: 8-10 / CALORIES: 390 / FAT: 33G / NET CARBS: 2G / PROTEIN: 20G

TOOLS

24 bamboo skewers

LAMB INGREDIENTS

2 pounds lamb, cut into 1½-inch cubes

Coarsely ground black pepper

Fresh sea salt

4 tablespoons extra-virgin olive oil

4 garlic cloves, crushed

2 teaspoons rosemary, finely chopped

1 teaspoon ground cumin

1 red onions, cut into square pieces

1 red peppers, cut into square pieces

MINT CHIMICHURRI INGREDIENTS

2 garlic cloves

2 cups flat-leaf parsley

2 cups mint leaves

1 small shallot

¼ small lime, juiced

4 tablespoons red wine vinegar

½ cup olive oil

Coarsely ground black pepper

Fresh sea salt

1. The night before you plan to grill, season the lamb cubes with coarsely ground black pepper and fresh sea salt. Set aside.

2. Next, in a large sealable plastic bag (if you need two, divide recipe between both bags), combine the remaining ingredients except for the onion and pepper. Add the lamb cubes to the bag and then transfer to the refrigerator, letting the meat marinate from 4 hour to overnight, the longer the better.

3. An hour and a half before grilling, remove the lamb from the refrigerator and let rest, uncovered and outside of the marinade, at room temperature.

4. In a small food processor, puree the garlic, parsley, mint, shallot, lime juice, and red wine vinegar. Slowly beat in the olive oil, and then remove from the processor. Season with coarsely ground black pepper and fresh sea salt, cover and then set aside.

5. A half hour before grilling, prepare your gas or charcoal grill to medium-high heat.

6. Pierce about four lamb cubes with each bamboo skewer, making sure to align the pieces of onion and pepper in between each cube.

7. When the grill is ready, at about 400 degrees with the coals lightly covered with ash, place the skewers on the grill and cook for about 15 to 20 minutes. Transfer the kebabs to a large carving board and let them rest for 5 minutes before serving with the Mint Chimichurri sauce.

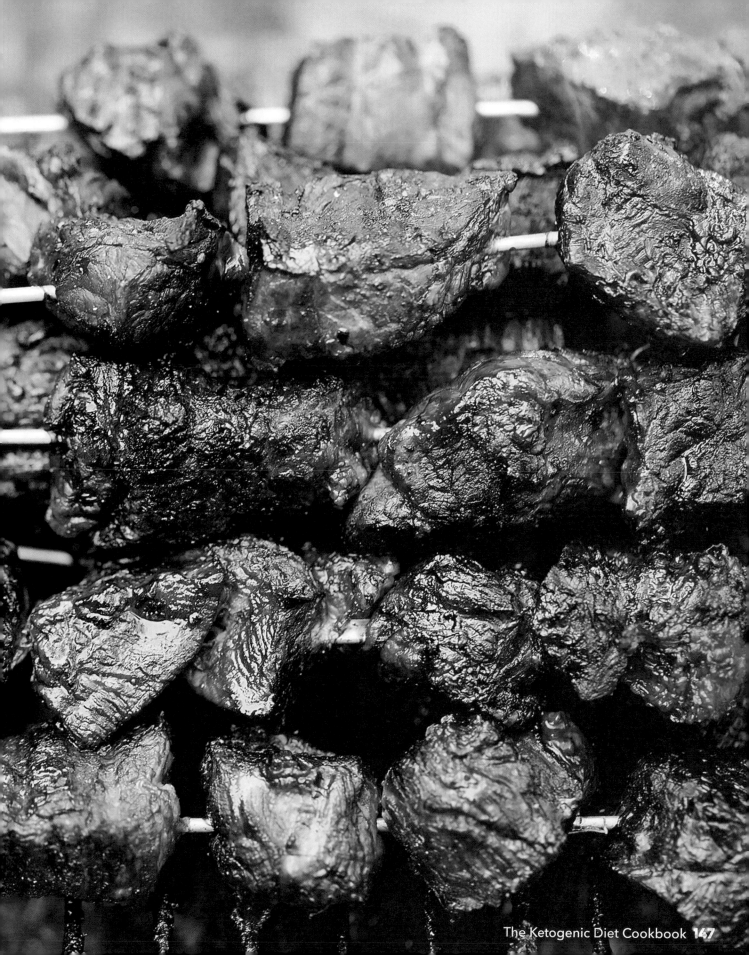

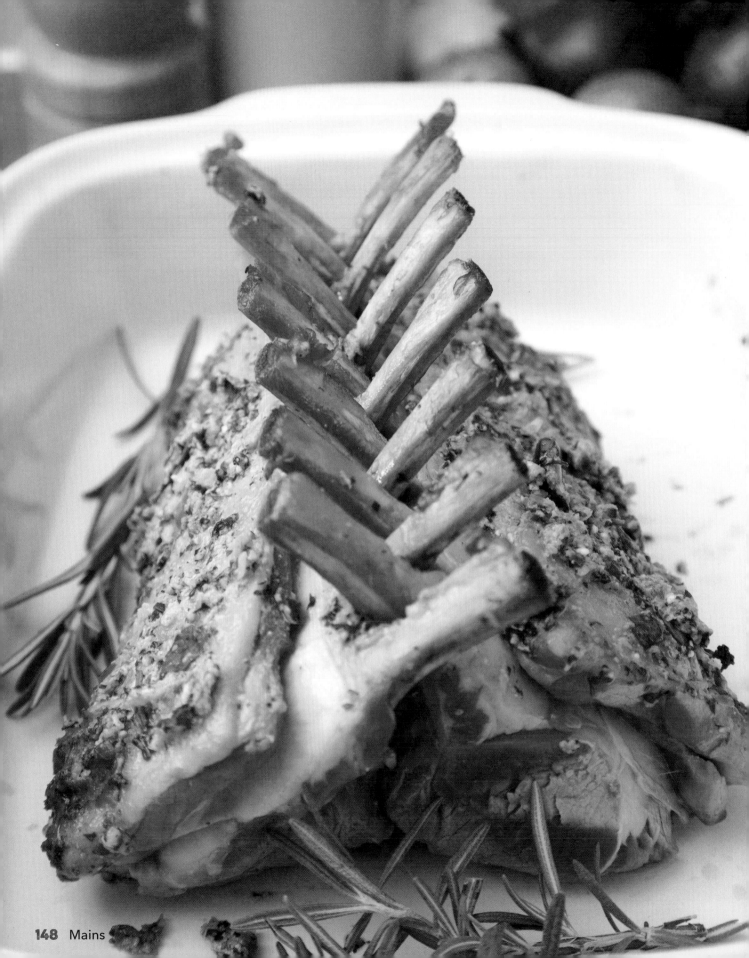

GRILL-ROASTED RACK OF LAMB WITH GARLIC-HERB CRUST

SERVES: 5-6 / CALORIES: 323 / FAT: 20G / NET CARBS: 3G / PROTEIN: 31G

2 tablespoons extra-virgin olive oil

2 garlic cloves, finely chopped

1 teaspoon lemon zest

Two 8-rib racks of lamb, about
1 pound each

Coarsely ground black pepper

Fresh sea salt

GARLIC-HERB CRUST INGREDIENTS

4 garlic cloves, finely chopped

½ small shallot, finely chopped

¼ cup flat-leaf parsley,
coarsely chopped

2 tablespoons rosemary, finely
chopped

1 tablespoon thyme, finely chopped

1 tablespoon olive oil

Coarsely ground black pepper

Fresh sea salt

1. The night before grilling, combine the olive oil, garlic, and lemon zest in a large sealable plastic bag. Pat dry the racks of lamb, and then season them with coarsely ground black pepper and fresh sea salt, kneading the pepper and salt deeply into the meaty sections of the lamb. Add the racks of lamb into plastic bag and place in the refrigerator. Let marinate overnight.

2. An hour and a half before grilling, remove the racks of lamb from the refrigerator and let rest, uncovered and at room temperature.

3. A half hour before grilling, prepare your gas or charcoal grill to medium heat.

4. While the grill heats, combine all of the ingredients to the garlic-herb crust in a small bowl. Next, take the racks of lamb and generously apply the crust ingredients to it, being sure to apply the majority of the crust on the meaty side of the rack.

5. When the grill is ready, at about 400 degrees with the coals are lightly covered with ash, place the meat-side of the racks of lamb on the grill and cook for about 3 to 4 minutes. When the crusts are browned, flip the racks of lamb and grill for another 5 minutes for medium-rare.

6. Transfer the racks of lamb from the grill to a large carving board and let rest for about 10 minutes before slicing between the ribs. Serve warm.

BIG TIP

Because the rack of lamb is a very delicate meat, be sure to give it the time to marinate overnight. I suggest pairing this with a glass of red wine.

CHICKEN CACCIATORE

SERVES: 6 / CALORIES: 263 / FAT: 13G / NET CARBS: 5G / PROTEIN: 27G

6 chicken breasts, skin removed (24 oz approx weight)

¼ cup extra-virgin olive oil

1 large onions, halved and thinly sliced

2 cloves garlic, minced

1 lb cremini mushrooms, wiped with a damp paper towel, trimmed, and sliced

14 oz can diced tomatoes, undrained

½ cup dry white wine

1 tablespoon fresh thyme

1 tablespoon fresh sage, chopped

1 tablespoon fresh rosemary, chopped

Salt and pepper to taste

1. Rinse chicken and pat dry with paper towels. Preheat the oven broiler, and line a broiler pan with heavy-duty aluminum foil. Broil chicken pieces for 3 minutes per side, or until browned. Transfer pieces to the slow cooker.

2. Heat oil in a large skillet over medium-high heat. Add onions, garlic, and mushrooms and cook, stirring frequently, for 5 minutes, or until mushrooms begin to soften. Scrape mixture into the slow cooker.

3. Add tomatoes, wine, thyme, sage, and rosemary to the cooker, and stir well. Cook on Low for 6 to 8 hours or on High for 3 to 4 hours, or until chicken is cooked through, tender, and no longer pink. Season to taste with salt and pepper.

BIG TIP

Most of the mushrooms we find in supermarkets are the same species, Agaricus bisporus. What makes the difference is their age. White button mushrooms are the youngest, cremini are in the middle, and Portobello is what we call them when they're big and old.

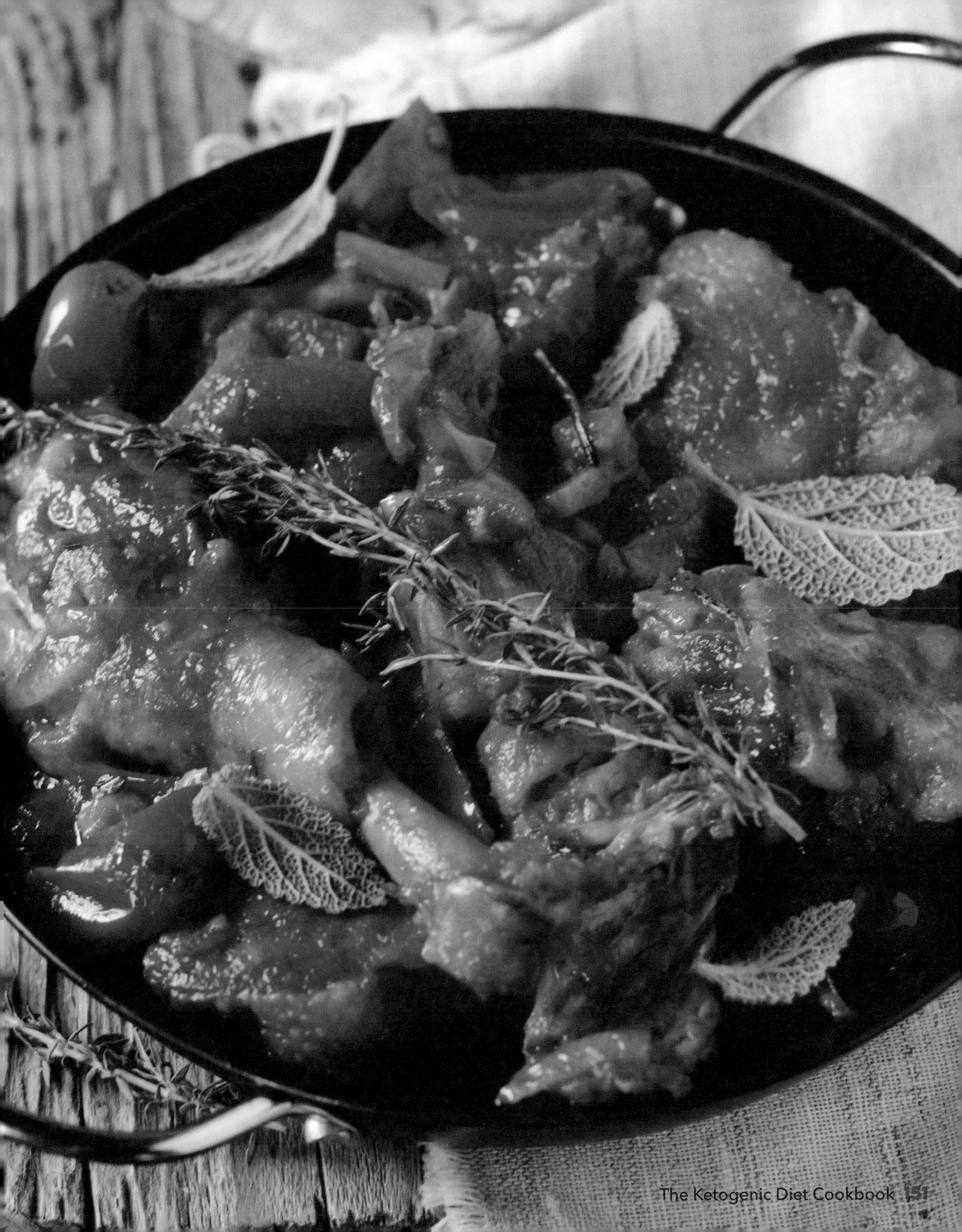

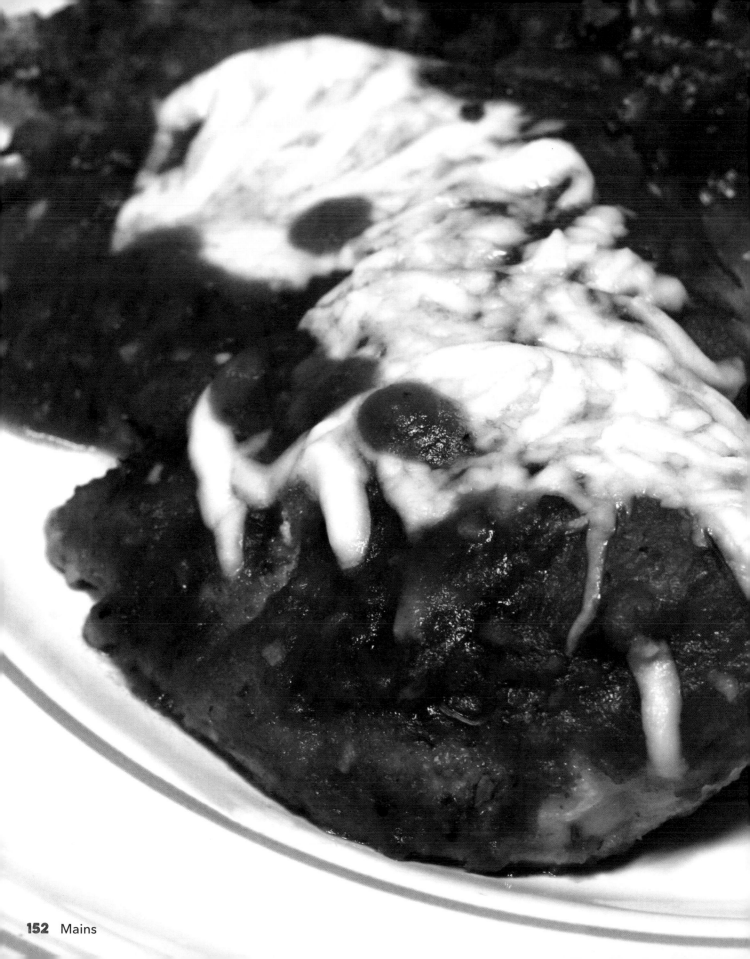

CHICKEN PARMESAN

SERVES: 4 / CALORIES: 388 / FAT: 22G / NET CARBS: 4G / PROTEIN: 45G

4 boneless, skinless chicken breasts (16 oz approx weight)

1 tsp garlic powder

Salt and pepper

1 tsp Italian seasoning mix

½ cup Parmesan cheese, grated

1 cup no-sugar spaghetti sauce (Prego and Classico are among the popular brands that make these)

8 ounces shredded mozzarella cheese

1. Place the chicken breasts in the slow cooker. Season by sprinkling over them the garlic powder, salt, pepper, Italian seasoning, and a generous shaking of Parmesan cheese. Pour the spaghetti sauce over the meat.

2. Cover and cook on Low for 6 hours or on High for 4 hours.

3. Uncover and top the chicken with the mozzarella cheese. Cover and continue to cook on Low for another hour or on High for another 30 minutes.

BIG TIP

Rather than sprinkle the meat with the seasonings, you can add them to your spaghetti sauce before pouring it on the chicken. You can also try a marinara sauce that has basil or red peppers, so long as there is no sugar added.

CHICKEN STUFFED WITH KALE AND CHEESE

SERVES: 4 / CALORIES: 389 / FAT: 22G / NET CARBS: 3G / PROTEIN: 38G

4 boneless, skinless chicken breasts (16 oz approx weight)

Salt and pepper for seasoning

¼ teaspoon dried oregano

½ teaspoon onion powder

½ teaspoon cayenne pepper

2 cups kale leaves, chopped

16 oz cheddar cheese cut into thick strips

Kitchen twine

½ cup dry white wine

1. The breasts should be on the thin side so they roll up easily. If they're thicker than ½ to ¼ inch, put them between pieces of waxed paper and use a meat mallet to pound them thin.

2. Sprinkle salt, pepper, oregano, onion powder, and cayenne on both sides of the cutlets. Put a layer of chopped kale in the center of each breast, lay a strip or so of cheese over to cover it, and top with some additional kale. Wrap the rolls tightly and secure with kitchen twine.

3. Lay the rolls in the slow cooker. Add the wine. Cover and cook on Low for 6 to 8 hours, or on High for about 5 hours, or until the juices run clear and the cheese is melted. If you want to "crisp" the outside, transfer the rolls to a foil-lined baking sheet and put them under the broiler for a few minutes.

BIG TIP

To add decadence to this recipe, cook 4 strips of bacon in the microwave until crispy, and add one to each roll before wrapping and securing the filling inside.

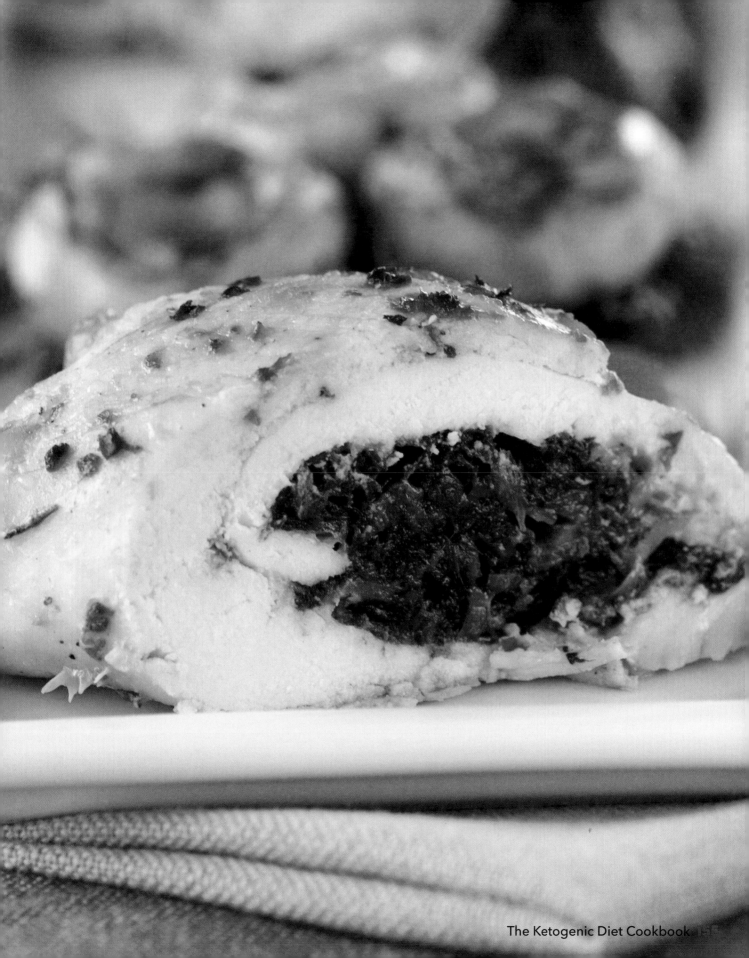

CORNISH HENS WITH FRESH GREENS

SERVES: 6 / CALORIES: 181 / FAT: 8G / NET CARBS: 3G / PROTEIN: 22G

---

2 tablespoons olive oil

1 small onion, minced

1 garlic clove, minced

2 small Cornish game hens, split in two, skin removed (20oz raw)

½ lbs Swiss chard, washed, coarse stems removed, and leaves chopped in large pieces

½ lbs Escarole, washed, trimmed, and chopped in large pieces

½ cup chicken stock or broth

1 lb baby spinach leaves

Salt and pepper to taste

1. Heat oil in a small skillet over medium-high heat, and cook onions and garlic about 3 minutes, or until onion is translucent. Scrape mixture into slow cooker.

2. Place Cornish hens on top of onion mixture, and top with Swiss chard, escarole, and stock.

3. Cover the slow cooker and cook on Low for 6 to 7 hours or on High for 3 to 4 hours, or until chicken is tender and cooked through.

4. Add the baby spinach and cook for another 20 to 30 minutes. Season with salt and pepper.

BIG TIP

The Cornish game hen is a young, immature chicken, which is technically not supposed to be over 5 weeks of age or more than 2 pounds. It's the result of crossing the Cornish game and Plymouth or White Rock chicken breeds.

BASIL CHICKEN BREASTS
WITH CHILE OIL

BASIL CHICKEN BREASTS SERVES: 4 / CALORIES: 172 / FAT: 7G / NET CARBS: 4G / PROTEIN: 23G
CHILE OIL SERVES: 12 / CALORIES: 120 / FAT: 14G / NET CARBS: 0G / PROTEIN: 0G

CHILE OIL INGREDIENTS

2 chile peppers of your choice

¾ cup olive oil

1 garlic clove, crushed

1 teaspoon ground coriander

CHICKEN INGREDIENTS

2 cups fresh basil leaves

3 scallions, chopped

2 garlic cloves

1 chile pepper of your choice, stemmed and coarsely chopped

¼ to ½ cup olive oil

4 skin-on boneless chicken breasts (4oz weight per breast)

Coarsely ground black pepper

Fresh sea salt

1. Add chile peppers into a small saucepan over medium-high heat. Lightly toast until the skin is blackened, about 3 to 4 minutes. Remove the chile and set aside. Next, add the 1/2 cup olive oil to the saucepan and heat. Mix in garlic and coriander and cook for 4 to 5 minutes. Then add the chile and cook for 4 more minutes. Remove and let rest overnight. (You can store the chile oil up to 4 months. Though, keep in mind that the longer the chile infuses into the oil, the hotter it will be!)

2. Mix the basil leaves, scallions, garlic, and chile pepper in a large bowl, and then add olive oil. Add the chicken breasts into the marinade and place in the refrigerator. Let soak for at least 4 hours or overnight.

3. Remove from the chile oil from the refrigerator and set aside. Also, transfer the chicken from the marinade to a large cutting board and let rest at room temperature for 30 minutes to 1 hour. Leave the marinade near the grill.

4. Prepare your gas or charcoal grill to medium-high heat.

5. When the grill is ready, at about 400 to 450 degrees with the coals lightly covered with ash, place the chicken on the grill and cook for about 7 minutes, frequently basting with the marinade. Flip and grill for another 5 to 6 minutes until finished; they should feel springy if poked with a finger.

6. Remove and let rest for 5 minutes. Serve warm with the chile oil drizzled on the side.

GRILLED GINGER SESAME CHICKEN

SERVES: 4 / CALORIES: 325 / FAT: 16G / NET CARBS: 2G / PROTEIN: 45G

2 tablespoons, plus ½ teaspoon extra-virgin olive oil

1- to 2-inch piece ginger, peeled and sliced

2 green onions, finely chopped

2 garlic cloves, minced

½ small lemon, juiced

4 boneless chicken breasts, (2lbs weight)

Coarsely ground black pepper

Fresh sea salt

3 tablespoons sesame seeds

1. Heat the extra-virgin olive oil in a small skillet over medium-high heat. When hot, add the ginger, onion, garlic, and lemon juice and sauté for about 2 to 3 minutes, or until the onions are translucent and the garlic is crisp but not browned. Remove from heat and transfer to a small bowl.

2. Rub the chicken breasts with pepper and salt and put them in a medium sealable plastic bag. Add the ginger-onion mixture and press around the chicken breasts. Seal and let rest at room temperature for 30 minutes.

3. Prepare your gas or charcoal grill to medium-high heat.

4. In a small dish, mix ½ teaspoon olive oil with sesame seeds. Set aside.

5. When the grill is ready, about 400 to 450 degrees with the coals lightly covered with ash, place the chicken on the grill and sprinkle the tops with half of the oiled sesame seeds. Grill the chicken breasts for about 7 minutes. Flip and season with the remaining sesame seeds, and then grill for 5 to 6 more minutes. When finished, they should feel springy if poked with a finger.

6. Remove and let rest for 5 minutes. Serve warm.

BIG TIP

Before filling the chicken's cavity with the garlic, thyme, and rosemary, heavily rinse the cavity with a couple cups of orange juice and salt—an easy way to really up the flavor and wow your guests!

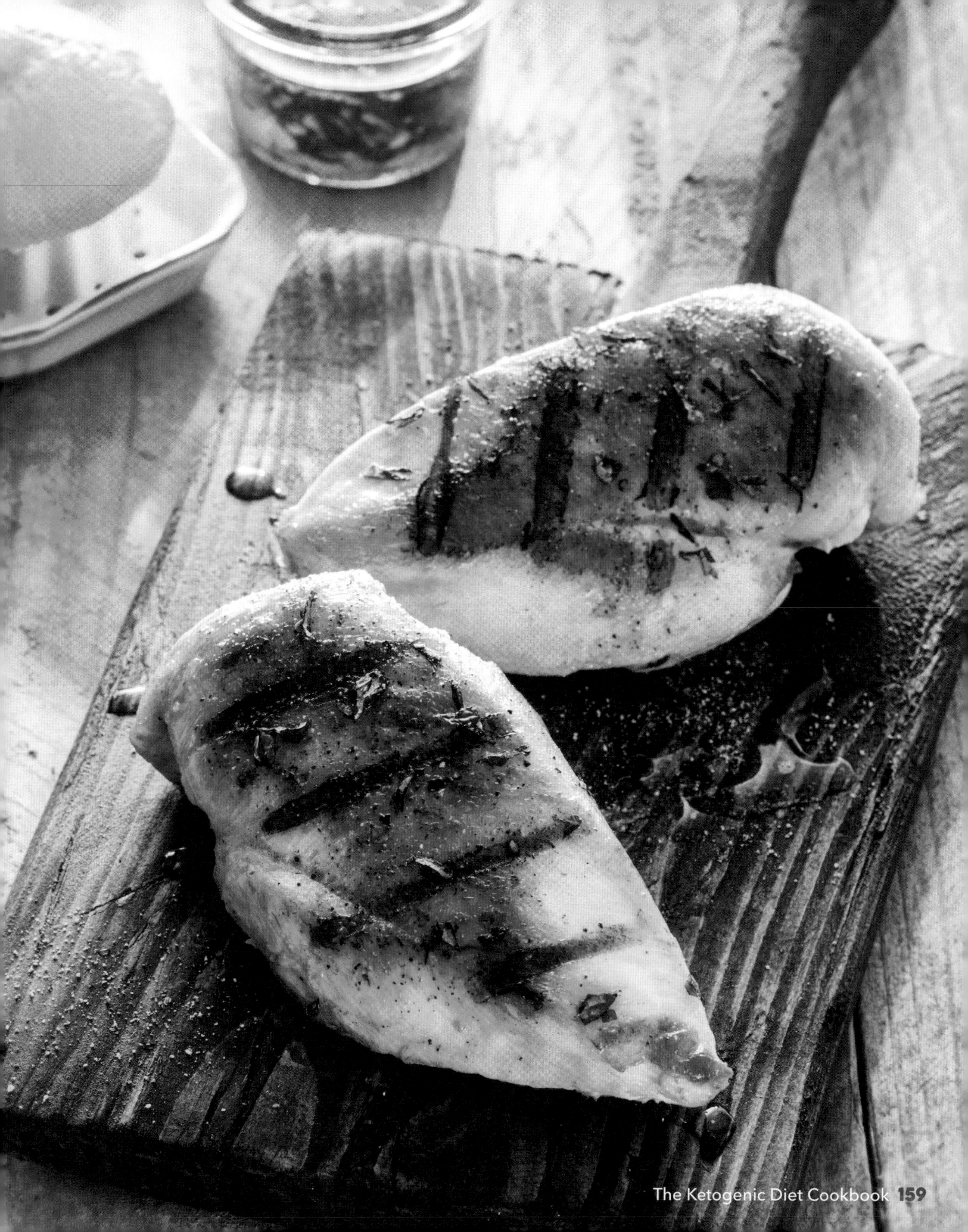

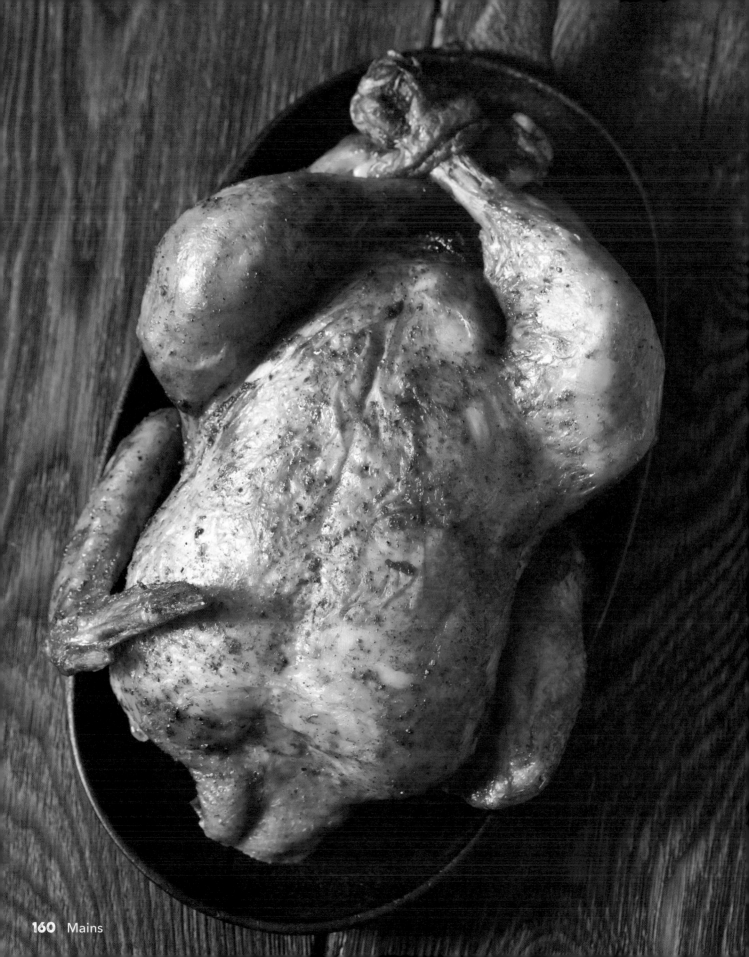

GRILLED LEMON AND GARLIC CHICKEN

CHICKEN BREAST SERVES: 4-5 / CALORIES: 228 / FAT: 9G / NET CARBS: 0G / PROTEIN: 35G
DRUMSTRICK AND THIGH CALORIES: 310 / FAT: 18G / NET CARBS: 0G / PROTEIN: 34G

TOOLS

1 to 2 feet butcher's twine

INGREDIENTS

A 4- to 5-pound chicken

Coarsely ground black pepper

Fresh sea salt

3 lemons, halved

1 garlic head, halved

1 bunch thyme

1 bunch rosemary

5 tablespoons extra-virgin olive oil

1. Prepare your gas or charcoal grill to medium heat.

2. Place the chicken into a large roasting pan and season its cavity generously with coarsely ground black pepper and fresh sea salt. Take 5 of the lemon halves and put them into the cavity, gently juicing them while doing so. Then, grab the remaining lemon half and rub it across the chicken, squeezing it lightly so that its juices seep into the chicken. Discard this half. Fill the cavity with the 2 halves of the garlic head and the thyme and rosemary, and tie the legs together with the butcher's twine. Let rest for 15 minutes.

3. Take 4 tablespoons of extra-virgin olive oil and massage it over the chicken's skin. Season the outside with additional pepper and salt.

4. When the grill is ready, at about 400 degrees with the coals lightly covered with ash, place the chicken on the grill, skin side up. Cover the grill and cook for about 40 minutes. Before flipping, brush the top of the chicken with the remaining tablespoon of olive oil. Turn and cook for about 15 more minutes until the skin is crisp and a meat thermometer, inserted into the thickest part of the thigh, reads 165 degrees.

5. Remove from grill and place on a large carving board. Let the chicken rest at room temperature for 10 minutes before carving. Serve warm.

POACHED POULTRY BREASTS

CHICKEN BREASTS SERVES: 6 / CALORIES: 96 / FAT: 14G / NET CARBS: 0G / PROTEIN: 4G
COOKING LIQUID CALORIES: 210 / FAT: 14G / NET CARBS: 14G / PROTEIN: 4G

6 chicken boneless, skinless chicken breasts (24 oz approx weight)

1 tablespoon extra-virgin olive oil

1 onion, chopped fine

2 cloves garlic, minced

2 cups chicken broth

2 cups water

Juice of ½ lemon

1 bouquet garni (see sidebar)

1 teaspoon whole white peppercorns

1. Place chicken breasts in the slow cooker.

2. Heat oil in a skillet and add the onions and garlic. Cook until the onions are translucent, 3 to 5 minutes. Transfer the onion mixture to the slow cooker. Cover the breasts with the chicken broth and water, and squeeze the lemon juice over everything. Add the peppercorns and the bouquet garni.

3. Cover and cook on Low for 8 to 10 hours or on High for about 7 hours. Remove the bouquet garni after 4 hours. Remove the cooked chicken with a slotted spoon, and allow to cool thoroughly. Put in a bowl covered with plastic wrap, and serve cold—perfect for chicken salad.

BIG TIP

The bouquet garni is a bundle of herbs traditionally used to flavor soups, stews, and sauces. While there's some variation, use the classic combination for this recipe. Take 2 sprigs of fresh thyme, 2 sprigs of parsley, and a large bay leaf. Tie the herbs together with kitchen string. This dish is quite low on fat so it's best to serve the chicken shredded in a salad with some homemade mayonnaise which is high in fat or a tablespoon of olive oil. The left over cooking liquid can work well in soups and stews.

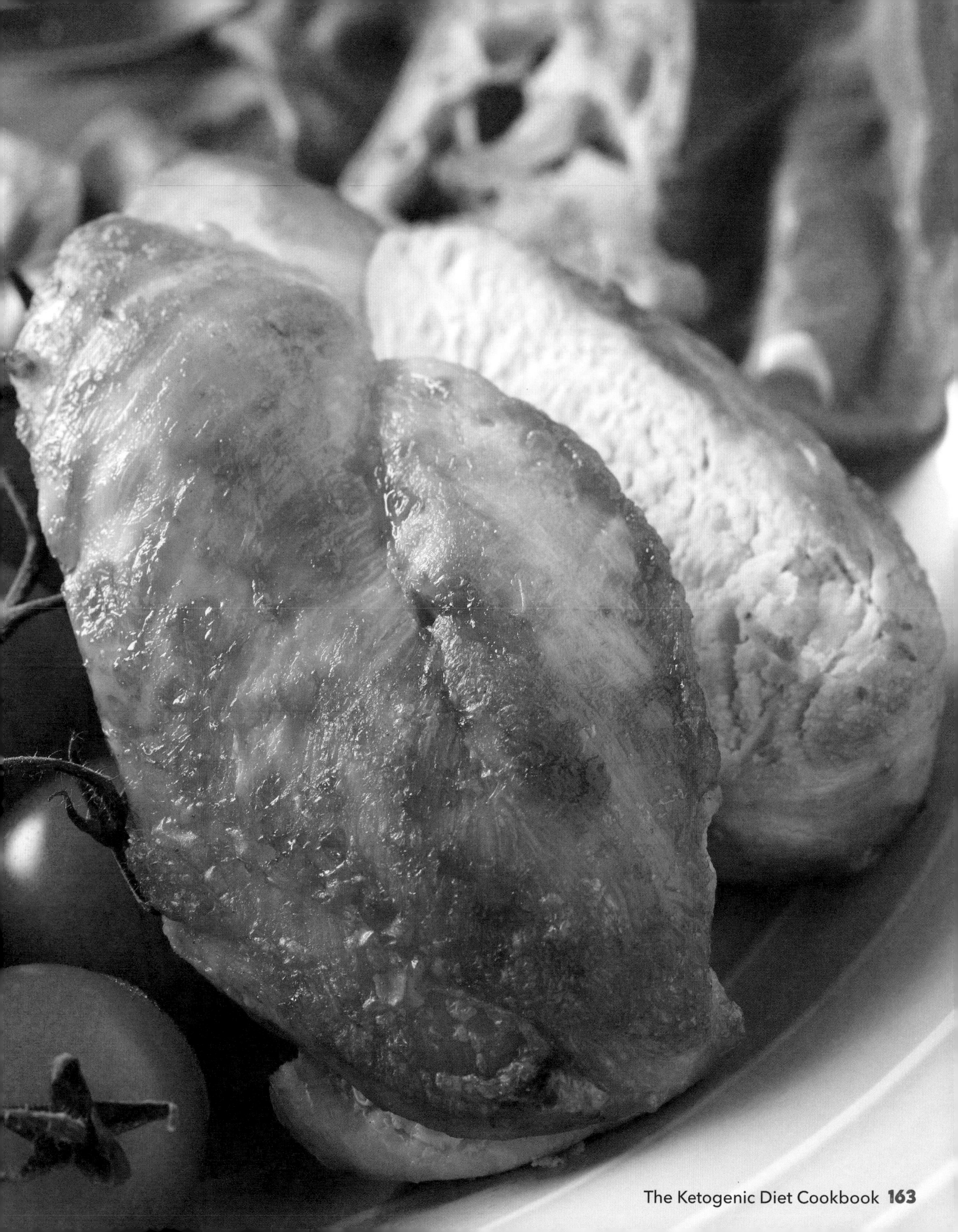

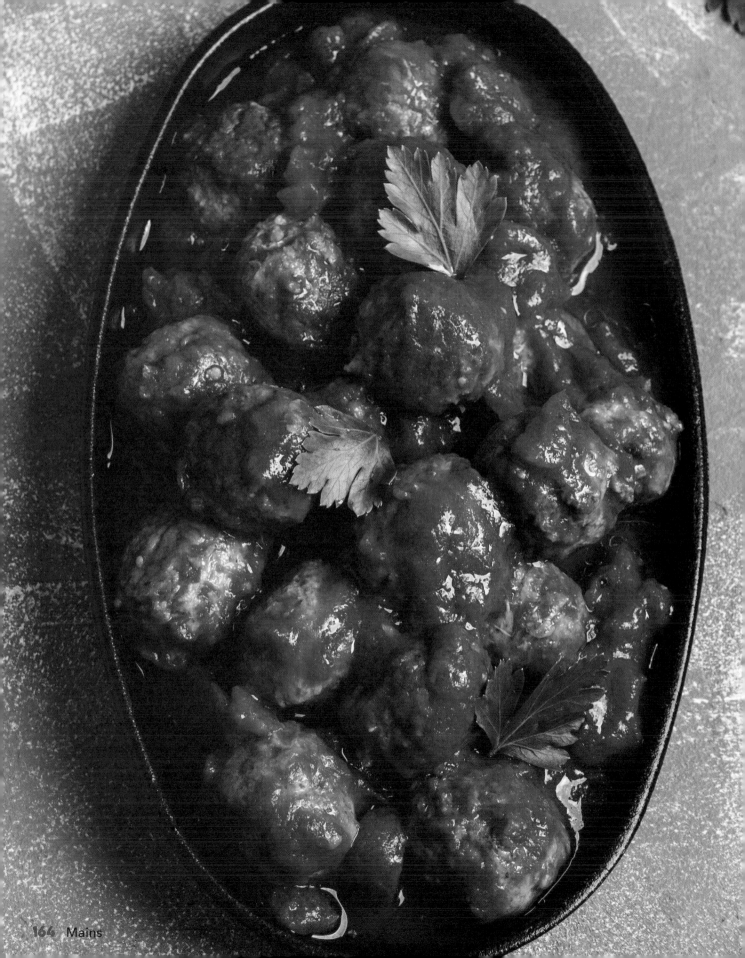

TURKEY MEATBALLS ON TOP OF ZUCCHINI

SERVES: 6 / CALORIES: 146 / FAT: 6G / NET CARBS: 5G / PROTEIN: 17G

1 lb ground turkey

1 egg

½ onion, minced

1 tablespoon fresh parsley, chopped fine

2 cloves garlic, put through a garlic press

Salt and pepper to taste

2 large zucchini, sliced thin

14 oz fresh pureed tomatoes

1. In a large bowl, combine the turkey, egg, onion, parsley, garlic, and a sprinkling of salt and pepper. Stir thoroughly.

2. Put the zucchini slices in the slow cooker. Form the meat into meatballs, and put them on top of the zucchini. Add the tomatoes over everything.

3. Cover and cook on Low for 4 to 6 hours or on High for 3 to 4 hours, until meatballs are cooked through and zucchini is tender. Season with additional salt and pepper if desired.

BIG TIP

Substitute any other kind of ground meat in this recipe. With the egg, onion, garlic, and parsley, you'll still fashion delicious meatballs. Vary the spices to create different flavor profiles. Add some heavy cream or butter over each serving for more fat.

MARYLAND CRABS

SERVES: 4 / CALORIES: 505 / FAT: 27G / NET CARBS: 0G / PROTEIN: 62G

2 cups water

½ cup distilled vinegar

¼ cup Old Bay Seasoning

1 tablespoon salt

Blue crabs (3 lbs total weight)

½ cup unsalted butter, melted

1. In a bowl, mix the water, vinegar, seasoning, and salt until well combined. Pour into the slow cooker. Cover and turn to High.

2. After 1 hour, add the crabs. Cover again and continue to cook on High for about 2 more hours, until crabs have turned bright red and cooked through.

3. Divide the butter into bowls for dipping.

BIG TIP

It's so worth the splurge to order Maryland blue crabs online. They arrive super-fresh and ready to cook and eat. What a treat!

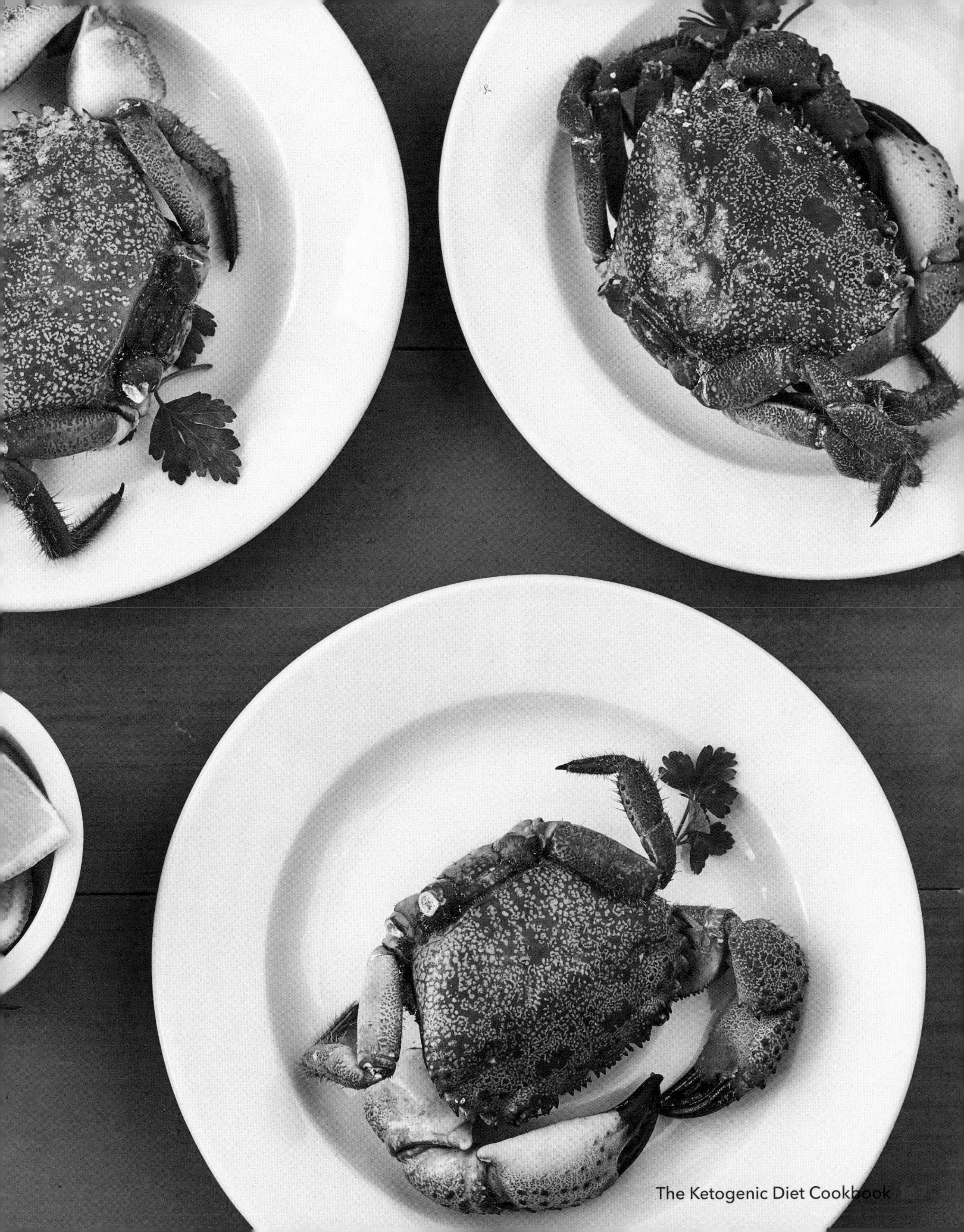

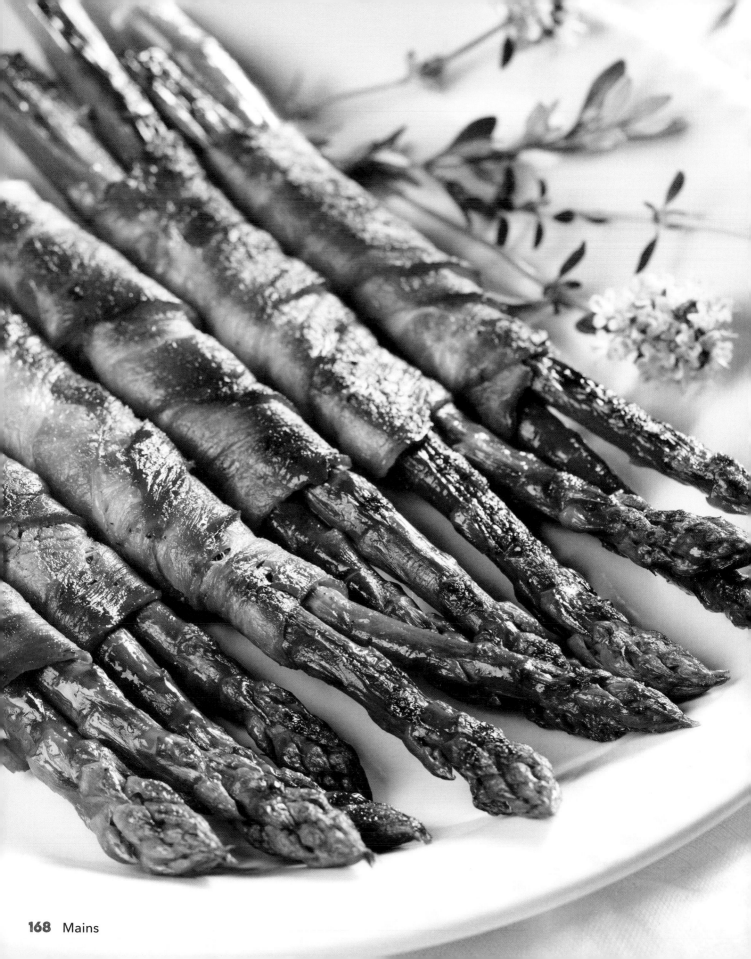

GRILLED FLOUNDER WITH BACON-WRAPPED ASPARAGUS

GRILLED FLOUNDER SERVES: 4 / CALORIES: 276 / FAT: 16G / NET CARBS: 2G / PROTEIN: 26G
BACON WRAPPED ASPARAGUS CALORIES: 344 / FAT: 38G / NET CARBS: 2G / PROTEIN: 3G

TOOLS

Handful of long toothpicks,
or 1 to 2 feet butcher's twine

4 sheets aluminum foil

FLOUNDER INGREDIENTS

4 large flounder fillets
(approx 24oz in total weight)

Coarsely ground black pepper

Fresh sea salt

4 tablespoons clarified butter

4 teaspoons dry white wine

2 garlic cloves, sliced

8 sprigs thyme

1 small lemon, sliced into wedges

BACON-WRAPPED ASPARAGUS

1½ pounds asparagus,

cut to 4-inch pieces

4 to 6 slices of thick bacon

2 tablespoons extra-virgin olive oil

Coarsely ground black pepper

1. Season the flounder fillets with coarsely ground black pepper and fresh sea salt and place each fillet on separate sheets of aluminum foil. Divide the clarified butter and dry white wine evenly across the fillets, and then do the same with garlic. Top each fillet with 2 sprigs of thyme, and then fold the bottom-half of the aluminum foil over the top, forming a tight crease along the side of the flounder.

2. Preheat your gas or charcoal grill to medium-high heat.

3. On a large carving board, arrange the asparagus into groups of 4 or 5. Spread the bacon strips apart, and then move each asparagus group onto the end of 1 strip of bacon. Pull the asparagus tightly together, piling some on top of the others, and then roll the bacon strip around it. When rolled tight, either pierce through the center with a long toothpick, or tie with butcher's twine. Set beside the grill.

4. When the grill is ready, at about 450 to 500 degrees with the coals lightly covered with ash, place the sealed flounder fillets on the grill and cover the grill and cook for about 9 minutes, flipping once, until the flounder fillets feel firm when poked with a finger. Transfer to a large carving board and let rest, their packets discarded, for 10 to 15 minutes.

5. While the flounder rests, place the bacon-wrapped asparagus on the grill and cook until the bacon and the asparagus are both charred, about 5 to 10 minutes.

6. Remove the bacon-wrapped asparagus from the grill and plate alongside flounder fillets. Garnish with wedges of lemon.

GRILL-SEARED LEMON HADDOCK
WITH BASIL-WALNUT PESTO

GRILLED HADDOCK SERVES: 4 / CALORIES: 277 / FAT: 15G / NET CARBS: 1G / PROTEIN: 33G
BASIL WALNUT PESTO CALORIES: 344 / FAT: 38G / NET CARBS: 2G / PROTEIN: 3G

HADDOCK INGREDIENTS

1½ pound Alaskan haddock fillets

¼ cup extra-virgin olive oil

Coarsely ground black pepper

Fresh sea salt

1 lemon, halved

BASIL WALNUT PESTO

½ cup walnuts

1 bunch basil leaves

1 tablespoon cilantro leaves

2 garlic cloves

½ cup olive oil

Coarsely ground black pepper

Fresh sea salt

1. Place the haddock fillets into a small baking pan and then add the olive oil. Season the fillets with coarsely ground black pepper and sea salt, then with freshly squeezed lemon juice. Let rest at room temperature while preparing the grill.

2. A half hour before cooking, place a cast-iron skillet on your gas or charcoal grill and prepare to medium heat. Leave the grill covered while heating, as it will add a faint smoky flavor to the skillet.

3. While the grill heats, puree the walnuts, basil, cilantro, and garlic cloves in a small food processor. When the mixture is a thick paste, slowly blend in the olive oil until you reach a consistency you like. Remove from food processor, season with black pepper and salt, and set aside.

4. When the grill is ready, at about 400 to 500 degrees with the coals lightly covered with ash, add the fillets into the skillet and sear for about 5 minutes. When the fillets have browned, turn and cook for 1 to 2 more minutes, until the fish is opaque through the center.

5. Transfer the haddock fillets to a carving board and let rest, uncovered, for 5 to 10 minutes. Serve with the basil walnut pesto.

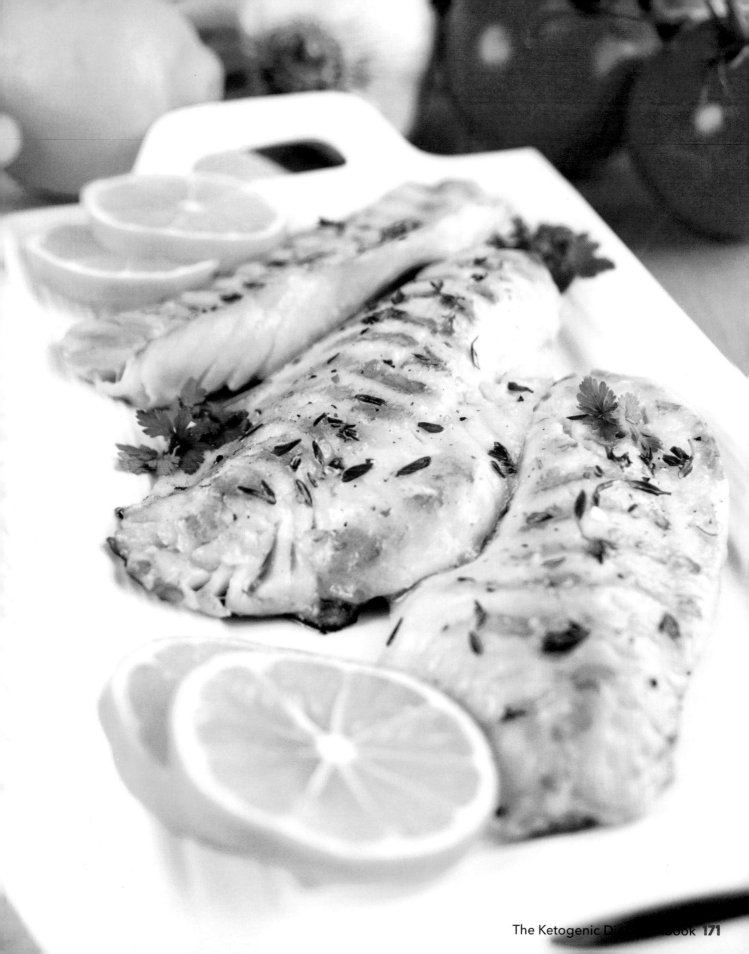

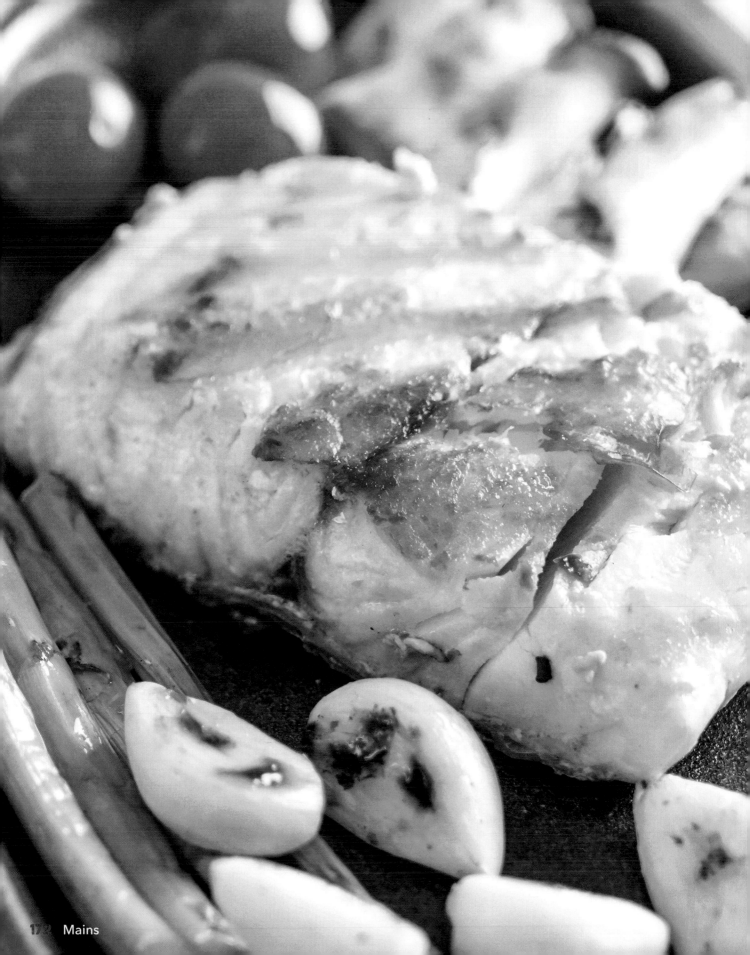

GRILLED RED SNAPPER
WITH CHILE-TOMATO SAUCE

GRILLED SNAPPER SERVES: 4 / CALORIES: 282 / FAT: 10G / NET CARBS: 1G / PROTEIN: 45G
SAUCE CALORIES: 93 / FAT: 7G / NET CARBS: 5G / PROTEIN: 1G

SNAPPER INGREDIENTS

4 red snapper fillets, skin-on and about 1½ to 2 inches thick

2 tablespoons olive oil

2 teaspoons red pepper flakes (optional)

Coarsely ground black pepper

Fresh sea salt

CHILE-TOMATO SAUCE INGREDIENTS

2 chile peppers of your choice

2 tablespoons olive oil

1 small shallot, finely chopped

2 garlic cloves, minced

16 oz large tomatoes, crushed

¼ cup fresh cilantro, finely chopped

1 tablespoon flat-leaf parsley, finely chopped

2 tablespoons fresh chives, finely chopped

Coarsely ground black pepper

Fresh sea salt

1. Rub the snapper fillets with olive oil and then season with the red pepper flakes, coarsely ground black pepper, and sea salt. Let stand at room temperature while preparing the grill and chile-tomato sauce.

2. A half hour before cooking, place a cast-iron skillet on your gas or charcoal grill and prepare to medium heat. Leave the grill covered while heating, as it will add a faint smoky flavor to the skillet.

3. When the grill is ready, at about 400 degrees with the coals lightly covered with ash, add the chile peppers and cook until the chiles are charred and wrinkled. Remove from pan and transfer to a small cutting board. Let cool and then stem the chiles. Finely chop them and set aside.

4. Add the olive oil to the cast-iron skillet. When hot, add the shallot and garlic cloves and cook until the shallot is translucent and the garlic is golden, about 2 minutes. Add the finely chopped chiles into the pan and sear for 1 minute. Mix in the tomatoes and cook until they have broken down. Stir in the cilantro, parsley, and chives and sear for a few more minutes. Season with the pepper and salt and transfer to a bowl. While the sauce is still hot, mash with a fork and cover with aluminum foil.

5. Place the seasoned snapper fillets on the grill directly over the heat source. Cover the grill and cook for about 3 minutes per side. When finished, the fillets should be opaque in the center and should easily tear when pierced with a fork. Transfer to a carving board and peel back the skin. Let rest 5 to 10 minutes, and then serve on beds of chile-tomato sauce.

SIMPLE SKILLET SALMON

SERVES: 4 / CALORIES: 521 / FAT: 31G / NET CARBS: 1G / PROTEIN: 57G

32 oz salmon filets

2 tablespoons unsalted butter, cut in pieces, softened

2 tablespoons extra virgin olive oil

1 lemon

Salt and pepper

1 tablespoon extra-virgin olive oil

1. Rinse the filets with cold water to ensure that any scales or bones are removed. Dry them in paper towels. Rub soft butter on both sides of the filets, squeeze lemon over them, and season with salt and pepper.

2. Heat the skillet over medium-high heat and add the tablespoon of extra-virgin olive oil and unused butter. Add the filets, flesh side down. Cook on one side for about 3 minutes, then flip them and cook only 2 minutes on the other side. Remove the pan from the heat and let the fish rest in it for a minute before serving. The skin should peel right off. Pour the oils from the pan over the fish before serving.

BIG TIP

There are different cuts of salmon: steaks and filets. The steaks are cut from the meat around the backbone, and they contain that bone in the middle. Filets are cut from the flesh that extends from the head to the tail of the fish. For this recipe, use filets.You can also toss some vegetables in the oil that remains in the pan after cooking the salmon for delicious sautéed veggies.

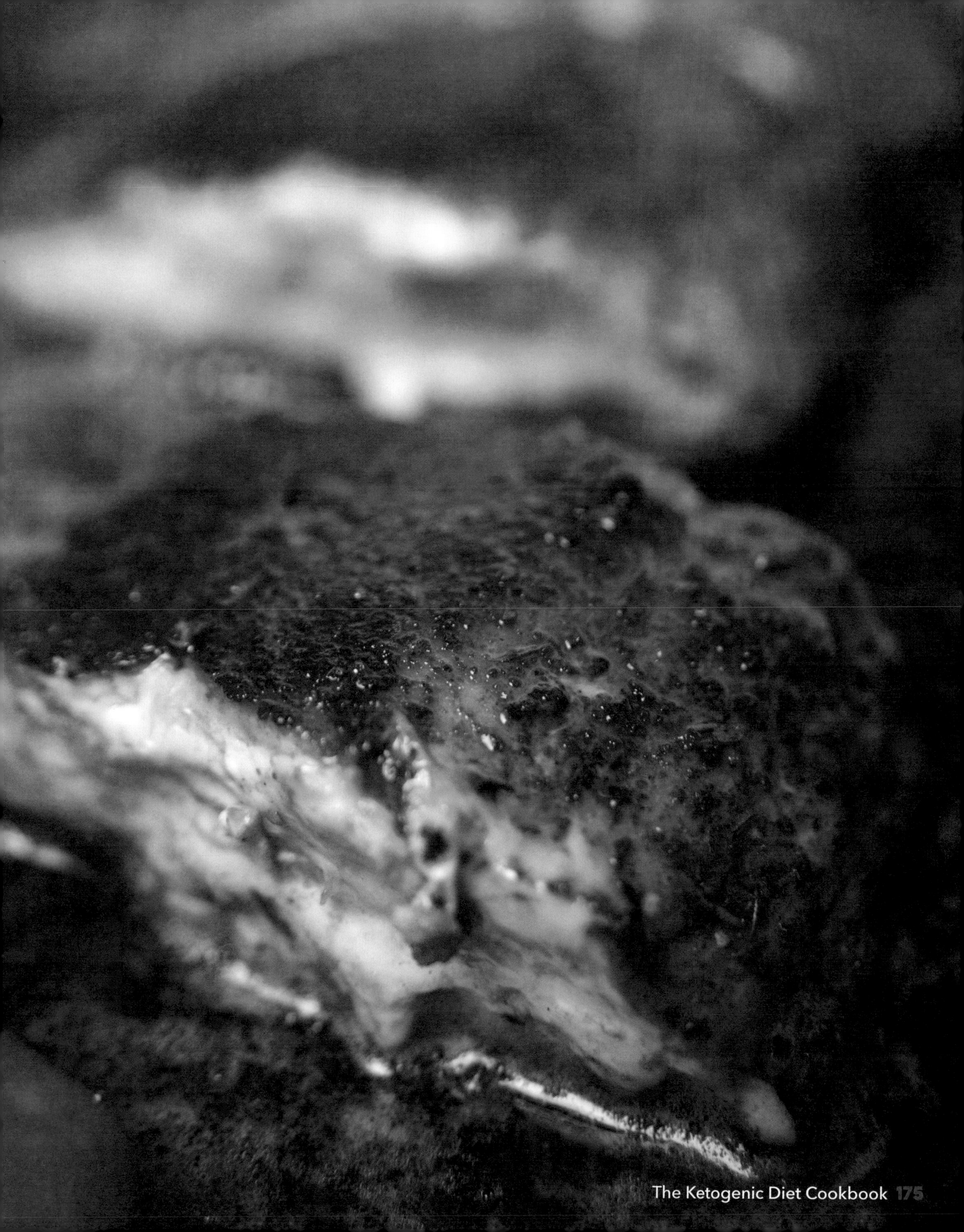

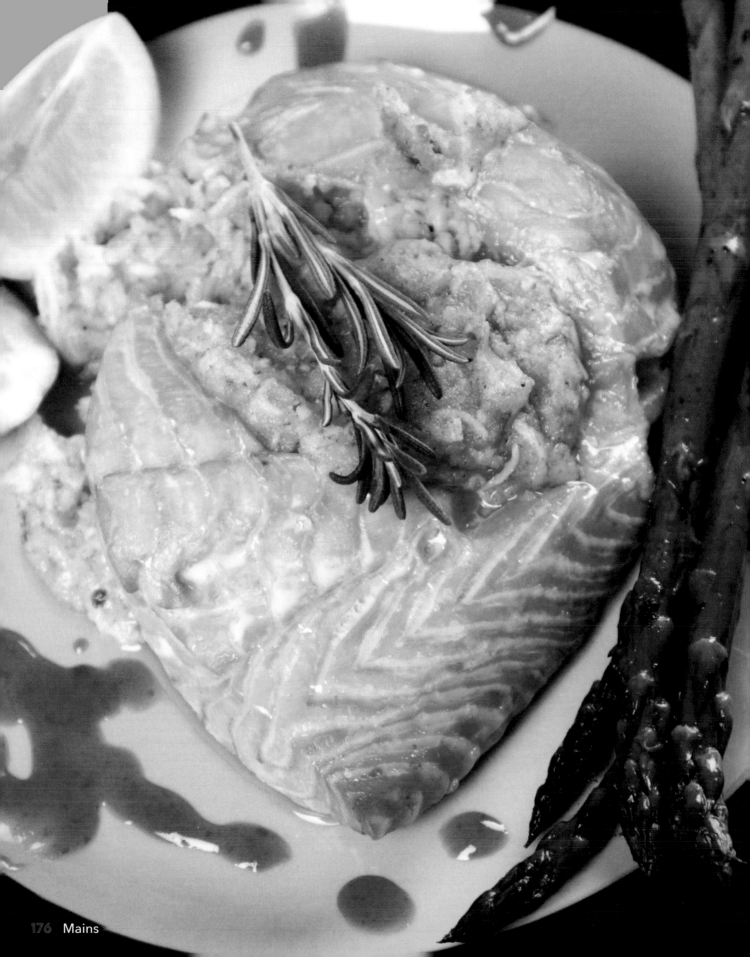

CRAB-STUFFED SALMON FILETS

SERVES: 6 / CALORIES: 415 / FAT: 23G / NET CARBS: 2G / PROTEIN: 51G

8 oz cooked crabmeat (fresh is best, but imitation will work), flaked

¼ cup celery, minced

2 cloves garlic, minced

¼ cup red pepper, minced

1 teaspoon fresh parsley, chopped fine

¼ teaspoon salt

½ teaspoon freshly ground pepper

1 teaspoon fresh lemon juice

1 egg

¼ cup unsalted butter, melted

6 salmon filets (about 6 oz each)

1. Make the crabmeat stuffing by combining the crabmeat, celery, garlic, red pepper, parsley, salt, pepper, lemon juice, egg, and melted butter in a bowl. Stir well to combine and make a nice stuffing mix.

2. Make a slit in the side of the salmon filets and evenly divide the stuffing into the filets. Gently transfer each stuffed filet to the slow cooker.

3. Cover and cook on Low for 4 to 5 hours until fish is cooked through.

BIG TIP

An excellent accompaniment to the stuffed salmon filets is spinach. Steam baby spinach leaves and make a pile of them in the center of a dinner plate. Place the stuffed salmon on top. Serve with lemon on the side. I'd splurge with a (small) glass of white wine!

SHRIMP SCAMPI

SERVES: 4 / CALORIES: 356 / FAT: 16G / NET CARBS: 3G / PROTEIN: 48G

2 lbs medium-sized raw shrimp, shells removed

2 tablespoons extra-virgin olive oil

2 tablespoons butter

4 cloves garlic, minced

1 tablespoon red pepper flakes

8 oz chopped tomatoes

2 cups water

1 teaspoon oregano

Salt and pepper to taste

1. Heat the oil and butter in a skillet and add the garlic, stirring until it sizzles. Add the tomatoes, red pepper flakes, oregano, salt, and pepper. Stir to combine and cook for about 3 minutes. Add in the water and bring to a boil.

2. Transfer sauce to the slow cooker. Place the shrimp on the sauce. Cover and cook on Low for 4 hours or on High for about 2 hours, until the shrimp are cooked through.

3. Serve straight out of the slow cooker with long forks or toothpicks.

BIG TIP

Make a meal out of this dish by serving the shrimp with the sauce over spaghetti squash. Not only will it be very tasty, the colors will be very nice.

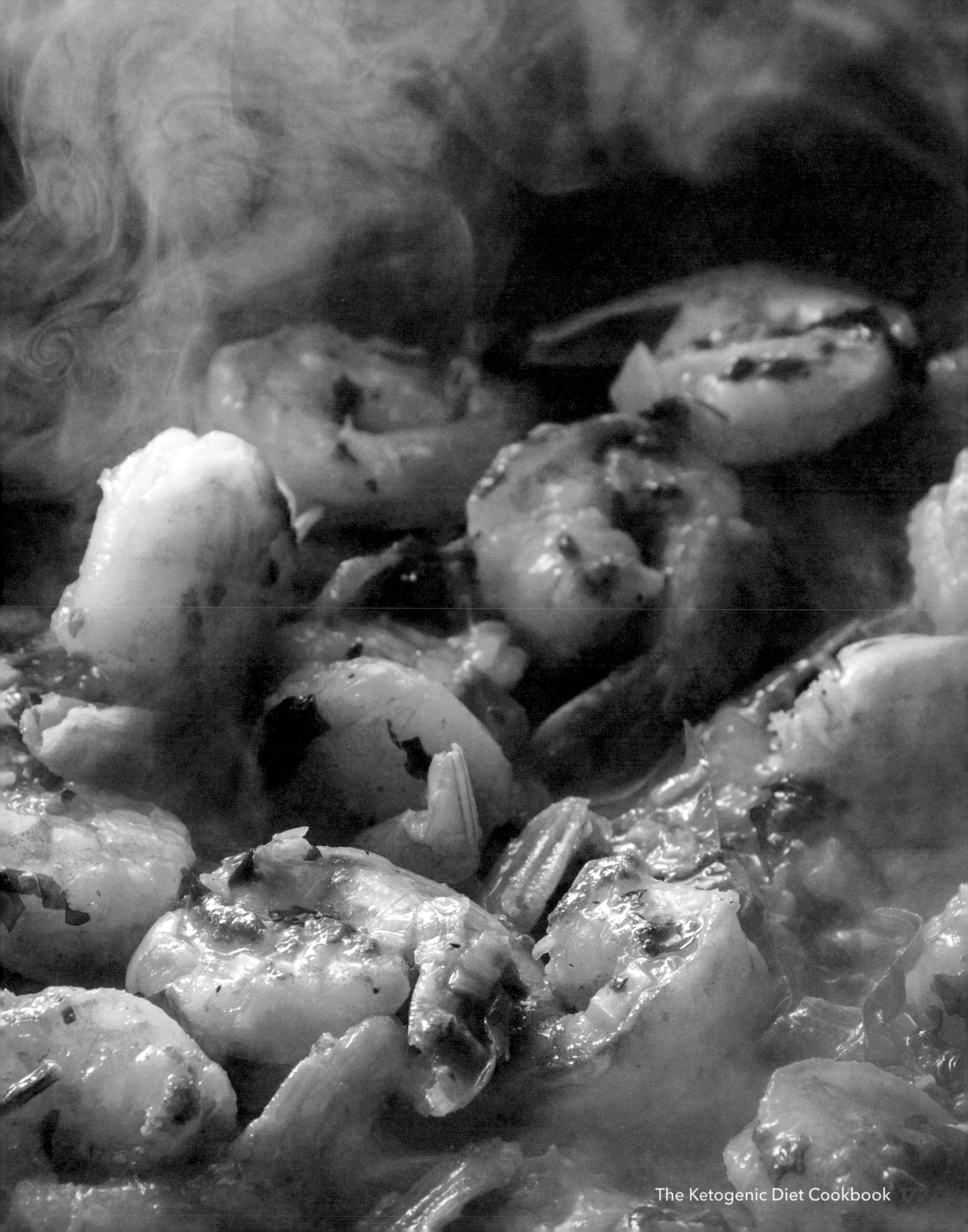

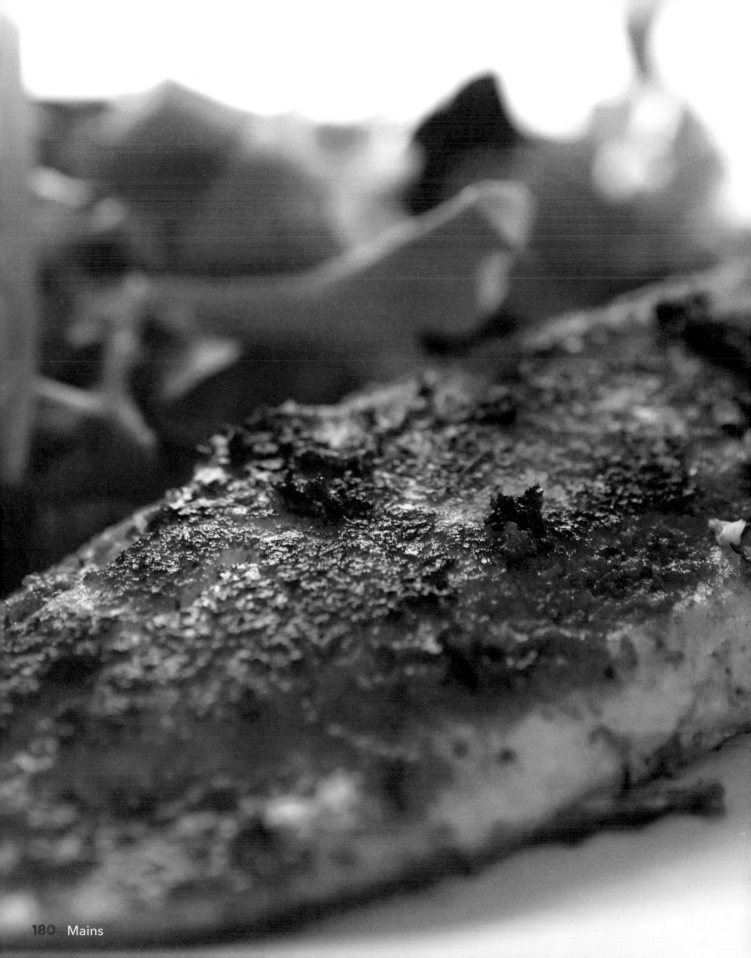

BLACKENED TILAPIA

SERVES: 4 / CALORIES: 378 / FAT: 4G / NET CARBS: 4G / PROTEIN: 21G

1 stick melted butter

4 boneless tilapia fillets, about 4 oz. each

1 lemon, cut into 4 wedges

BLACKENED SEASONING

1 tablespoon paprika

1 tablespoon onion powder

1 tablespoon garlic powder

2 tablespoons cayenne pepper

1 tablespoon white pepper

1 tablespoon finely ground black pepper

1 tablespoon dried thyme

1 tablespoon dried oregano

1. In a bowl, combine all the spices for your blackened seasoning and set aside.

2. Heat the skillet over high heat for about 10 minutes until very hot. While the skillet heats, rinse the fillets and then pat dry with paper towels. Dip the fish fillets in the melted butter, covering both sides, and then press the blackened seasoning generously into both sides.

3. Put the fish in the skillet and cook for about 3 minutes a side, placing a bit of butter on the tops while the bottoms cook. Serve with lemon.

BIG TIP

Tilapia is a wonderful fish for blackening, as it is a firm-fleshed fish that is fairly bland and thus benefits from seasoning. You can blacken any kind of fish, though. Others that taste great prepared this way are catfish, tuna, grouper, halibut, trout, and even shrimp.

SEARED TUNA STEAKS WITH DILL AIOLI

SERVES: 4 / CALORIES: 547 / FAT: 50G / NET CARBS: 1G / PROTEIN: 26G

TUNA STEAKS INGREDIENTS

4 fresh tuna steaks, about 2 inches thick

2 tablespoon extra-virgin olive oil,

plus a little extra for the grill

Coarsely ground black pepper

Fresh sea salt

DILL AIOLI INGREDIENTS

10 sprigs dill, finely chopped

10 sprigs parsley, finely chopped

¼ small lemon, juiced

1 garlic clove, minced

¾ cup olive oil

Fresh sea salt

1. Rub the tuna steaks with a little extra-virgin olive oil and then season with pepper and salt. Let rest at room temperature while you prepare the grill and basil aioli.

2. Prepare your gas or charcoal grill to high heat.

3. While waiting for the grill, combine the dill, parsley, lemon juice, and garlic clove into a small bowl and whisk together. While whisking, slowly incorporate the olive oil and season with fresh sea salt. Set aside or chill in the refrigerator. (If you want a lighter aioli, combine the initial ingredients in a blender and then slowly add the olive oil.)

4. When the grill is ready, at about 450 to 500 degrees with the coals lightly covered with ash, brush the grate with a little olive oil. Tuna steaks should always be cooked between rare and medium-rare; anything over will be tough and dry. To accomplish a perfect searing, place the tuna steaks directly over the hot part of the coals and sear for about 2 minutes per side. The tuna should be raw in the middle (cook 2½ to 3 minutes per side for medium-rare).

5. 5. Transfer the tuna steaks to a large carving board and let rest for 5 to 10 minutes. Slice against the grain and then serve with the dill aioli to the side.

BIG TIP

Seared tuna steaks are always a great on a warm summer evening. When serving these steaks, you have the option of serving chilled or right off the grill. The dill aioli is perfect when served slightly chilled. I recommend serving the steaks with the dill aioli and a side of grilled red peppers.

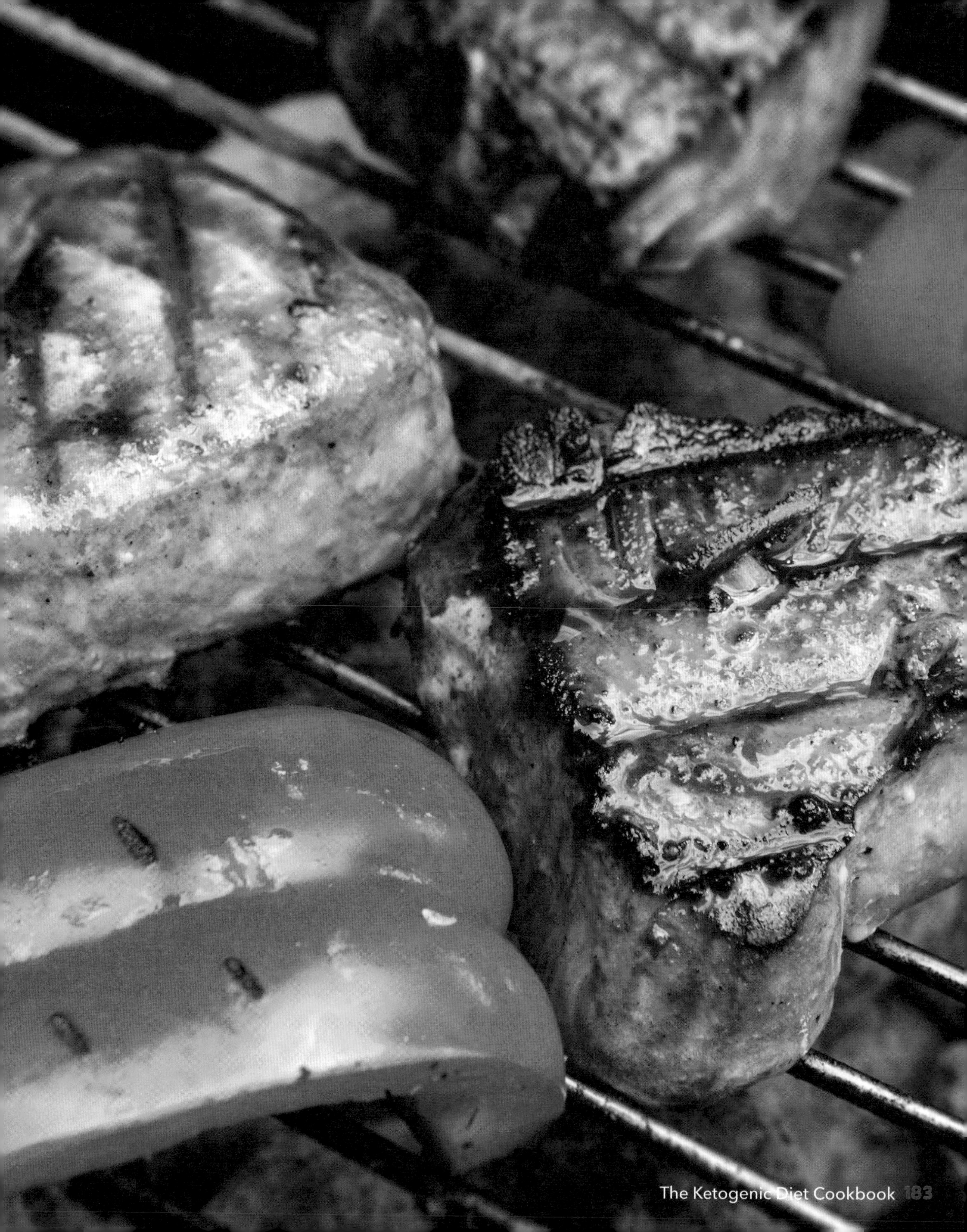

LEMON-TARRAGON BLUEFISH

SERVES: 4 / CALORIES: 545 / FAT: 26G / NET CARBS: 4G / PROTEIN: 69G

3 lbs bluefish fillet

2 tablespoons fresh tarragon,chopped

2 lemons

1 medium onion, thinly sliced

4 tbsp butter

Salt and pepper to taste

1. Make sure the fillets are free of bones. Put them skin side down into the slow cooker.

2. Sprinkle the tarragon over the fish, then squeeze the lemons over them. Remove any seeds. Thinly slice one of the squeezed lemons, and place the slices on the fish. Finally, top with the onion slices and butter.

3. Cook on Low for 3 to 4 hours or on High for 1 to 2 hours, until fish is cooked through and flakes easily.

BIG TIP

This simply prepared fish is also delicious chilled and served in lettuce wraps. Garnish with chopped cucumbers, cherry tomatoes, and a thin slice of avocado.

EGGPLANT ROLLATINI

SERVES: 4 / CALORIES: 508 / FAT: 42G / NET CARBS: 15G / PROTEIN: 15G

3 regular eggplants (about 8 inches)

½ cup extra-virgin olive oil

1½ cups ricotta

Zest of ½ lemon

1 tablespoon basil, chopped

Nutmeg, freshly grated

Parmesan cheese, to taste

Pinch of salt and pepper, to taste

1. Slice eggplant lengthwise to yield 12 slices. Place the slices in a colander and salt them.

2. After letting the slices drain for 20 minutes, dry and coat them in olive oil, salt and pepper.

3. Preheat grill to medium heat. Grill the slices for 10 minutes, flipping them over halfway through. Cook your slices until grill marks appear and they become slightly tender. Remove from heat and allow them to cool.

4. In a medium-sized bowl, mix together the ricotta, lemon zest, basil, nutmeg and as much Parmesan as you want.

5. Once everything is properly mixed, lay out your eggplant slices. Add a few tablespoons of the mixture to the end closest to you. Roll up the eggplant and secure it with a toothpick.

6. Grill the eggplant for about 2 more minutes, remove from heat and serve.

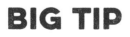

BIG TIP

ADD MEAT! Bacon bits make a great addition to your cheesy spread.

EGGPLANT RATATOUILLE

SERVES: 4-6 / CALORIES: 133 / FAT: 10G / NET CARBS: 6G / PROTEIN: 3G

1 cup brown rice

1 medium eggplant

1 medium summer squash

1 medium zucchini

1 medium onion

1 can stewed tomatoes

¼ cup parsley

¼ cup basil leaves

3 tablespoons olive oil

2 cloves garlic, minced

Pinch of dried basil, oregano,

salt and pepper

1. Cook brown rice according to package directions. Prepare vegetables by cutting eggplant into 1/2-inch pieces, the summer squash and zucchini in half lengthwise, and onions into quarters. Wash the eggplant pieces and sprinkle with salt. Let sit for 30 minutes.

2. In a large bowl, pour 2 tablespoons of olive oil. Add eggplant, squash, zucchini and onion to the bowl and toss to coat. Preheat grill to medium-high heat. Place eggplant, squash, and zucchini directly on the grill. Skewer the onions before placing on the grill. Grill vegetables until they are lightly charred: about 10-12 minutes for the onions, and 4-5 minutes per side for the eggplant, squash, and zucchini. Remove from heat and let cool.

3. Cut the eggplant into cubes and the squash and zucchini into slivers. Add 1 tablespoon of olive oil to a large saucepan and then cook over low heat until the garlic is golden, about 2 minutes. Stir in the grilled vegetables, stewed tomatoes, parsley, dried basil, oregano, salt and pepper. Cook for about 30 minutes. Stir in the basil leaves and then serve over brown rice.

BIG TIP

ADD MEAT! Sear pieces of top round beef cut into bite-sized pieces brushed in extra-virgin olive oil until they become golden brown. Add this to the saucepan.

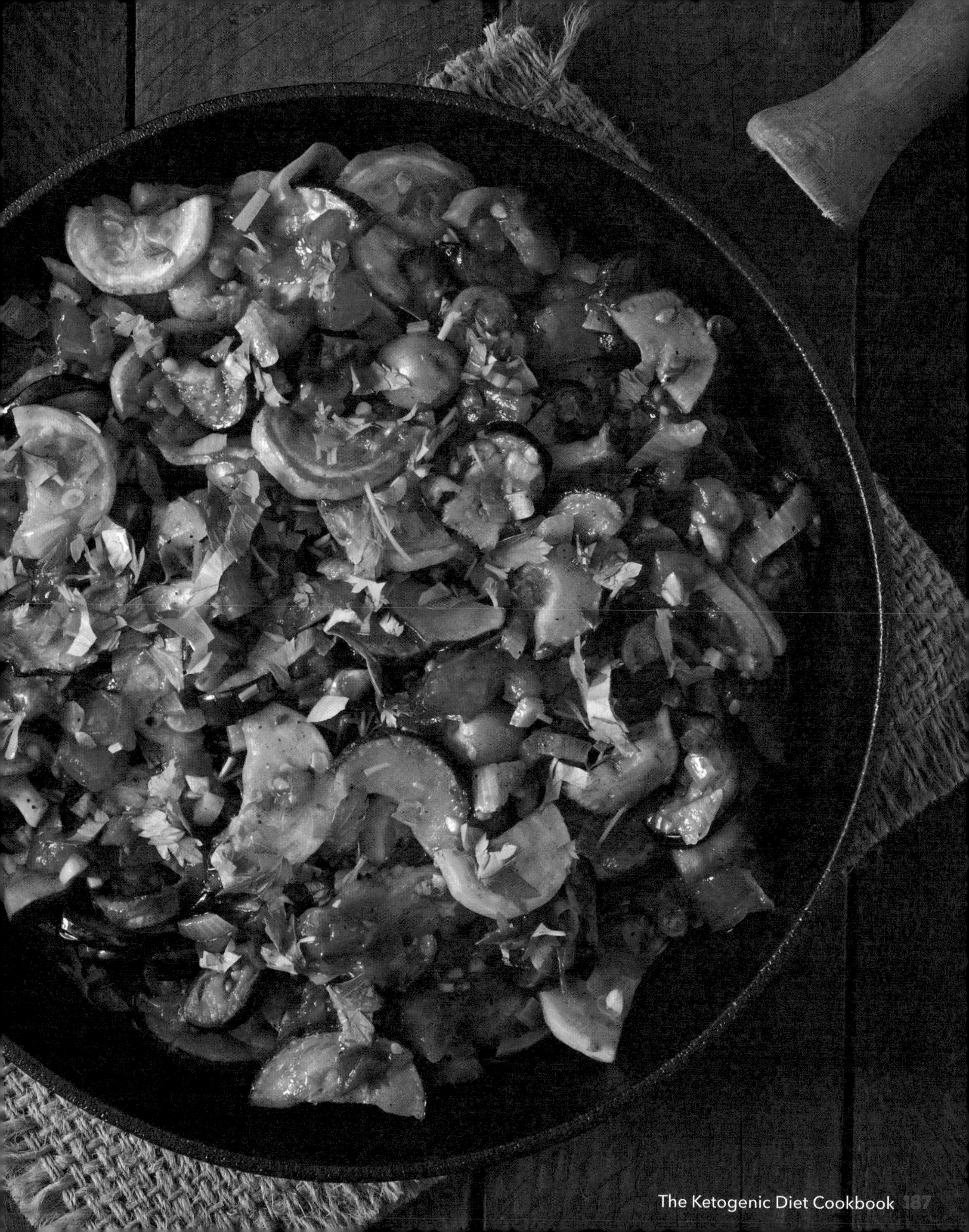

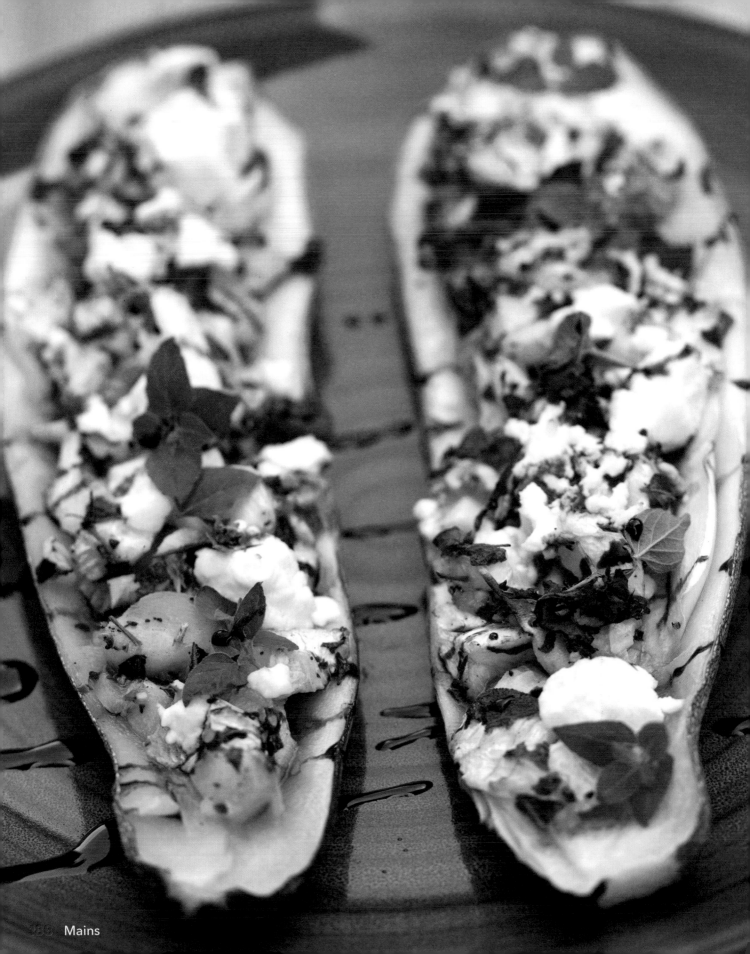

STUFFED ZUCCHINI

SERVES: 4 / CALORIES: 353 / FAT: 24 / NET CARBS: 9G / PROTEIN: 23G

4 medium-sized zucchini

15 ounces goat cheese

2 cups marinara sauce

Salt and pepper, to taste

1. Preheat your grill to high heat. Slice your zucchini in half, lengthwise. Hollow out the zucchini by removing seeds, creating a trough. Season the halves with a little salt and pepper.

2. Evenly spread the goat cheese in the troughs of each zucchini, using as little or as much as you'd like. Repeat the process with the marinara sauce.

3. Grill the logs until the cheese becomes soft and the marinara is bubbling slightly. This should take about 10 minutes. Remove from heat and serve.

BIG TIP

ADD MEAT! Add chopped up ham to the zucchini log when you add the goat cheese. Use a homemade marinara sauce for less carbs and add a tablespoon of butter before serving for more fat.

GRILLED ZUCCHINI PARM

SERVES: 4 / CALORIES: 347 / FAT: 27G / NET CARBS: 5G / PROTEIN: 21G

3 medium zucchini

2 tablespoons olive oil

2 tablespoons butter, softened

2 cloves garlic, minced

1 tablespoon parsley, chopped

½ cup Parmesan cheese, grated

Salt, to taste

1. Preheat grill to medium-high heat. Oil the grill to prevent sticking. Cut each zucchini lengthwise into four pieces. In a small bowl, mix together the olive oil, butter, garlic and parsley. Add a pinch of salt to the mixture, to taste. Use this mixture to coat the zucchini slices. Place these on the hot grates and grill until the slices are tender. This should take about 8 minutes. Sprinkle one side of the zucchini with Parmesan cheese. Remove from heat and serve.

BIG TIP

ADD MEAT! Add chicken or use it as a replacement for the zucchini. Coat 1 pound of skinless, boneless chicken in the same way you'd coat the zucchini and grill for 5-6 minutes per side, or until it is completely cooked through. Top with mozzarella cheese and cook until cheese melts.

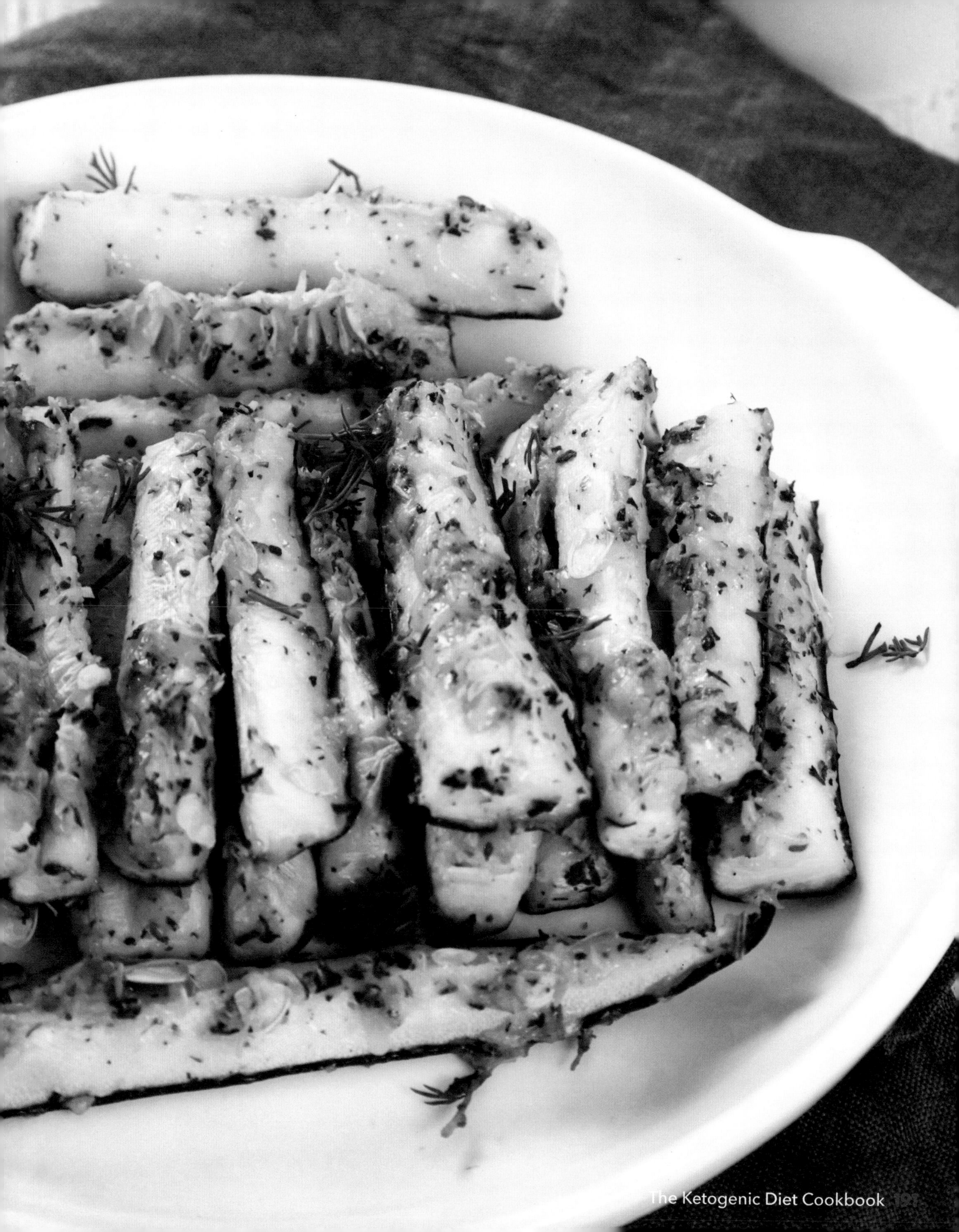

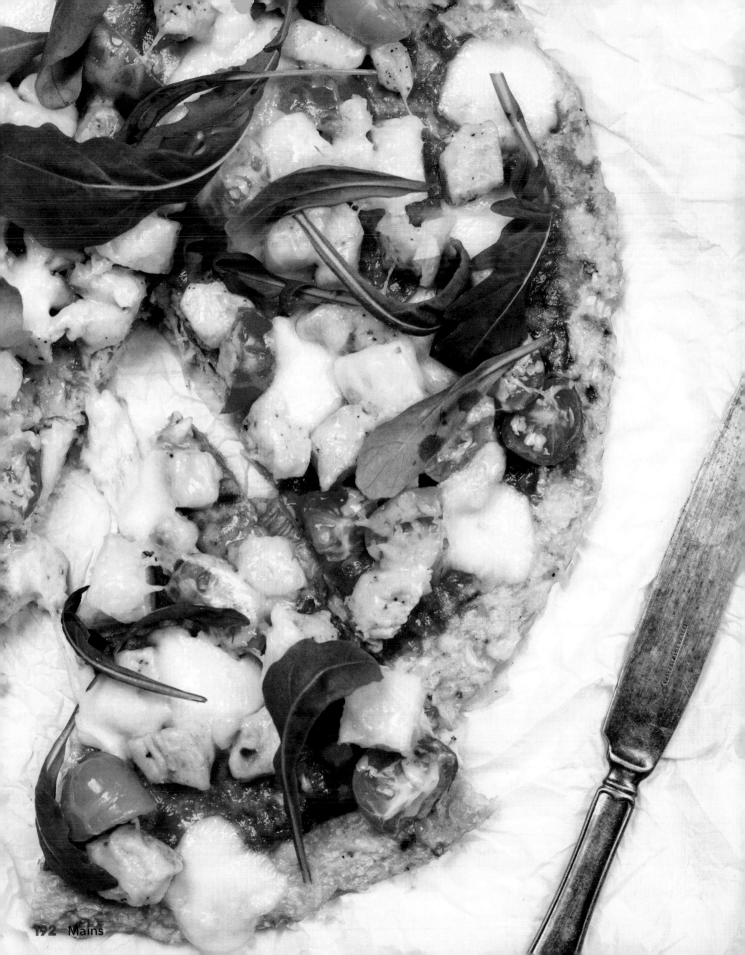

CAULIFLOWER GLUTEN-FREE PIZZA DOUGH

SERVES: 4 / CALORIES: 326 / FAT: 21G / NET CARBS: 4G / PROTEIN: 29G

1 standard bag of frozen cauliflower (12 oz)

¼ cup parmesan cheese, grated

2 cups mozzarella, shredded

3 teaspoons oregano

1 teaspoon basil

½ teaspoon salt

1 clove garlic, minced

2 eggs, lightly beaten

1. Steam the cauliflower according to the directions on the package. Cook the cauliflower ahead of time and let it dry overnight on a sheet pan in the refrigerator, or let it cool and pat dry. This will help get all of the water out and keep the crust as crisp as possible.

2. Pulse the completely dry cauliflower in a food processor and add it to a large bowl.

3. Add the Parmesan, mozzarella, oregano, basil, salt, garlic and eggs. Mix well and transfer mixture to a baking sheet.

4. Spread it into a large circle and bake for 20 minutes. After adding your pizza toppings, cook for another 10 minutes on the grill over medium heat!

BIG TIP

This pizza dough is perfect for anyone following a gluten-free diet. Just make sure the cauliflower is completely dry before processing it.

GRILLED EGGPLANT "PIZZAS"

SERVES: 4 / CALORIES: 295 / FAT: 23G / NET CARBS: 11G / PROTEIN: 7G

3 pounds eggplant

3 tablespoon salt

⅓ cup extra-virgin olive oil

Pinch of ground pepper

½ cup mozzarella cheese

1 cup low carb pizza sauce

Parmesan cheese

1. Cut your eggplant into ½-inch slices, sprinkling salt on both sides of every slice. Place the slices in a colander over your sink or a bowl. Let this stand for one hour to drain. Rinse the slices under cold water and place on several layers of paper towels to press the water out.

2. Preheat your grill to medium-high heat. Brush both sides of the slices with olive oil and sprinkle with some ground pepper. Place your slices on the grill and cook one side until it is slightly browned, taking 5-6 minutes.

3. Once that first side has cooked, flip the slice over and remove from heat to add sauce and cheese. Distribute sauce and mozzarella cheese over the grilled side of the slice.

4. Place eggplant back on the grill to cook the other side and melt the cheese. Remove from grill, top with Parmesan cheese and serve.

BIG TIP

ADD MEAT! Grill up a few slices of prosciutto and tear the slices, spreading evenly across the eggplant pizza.

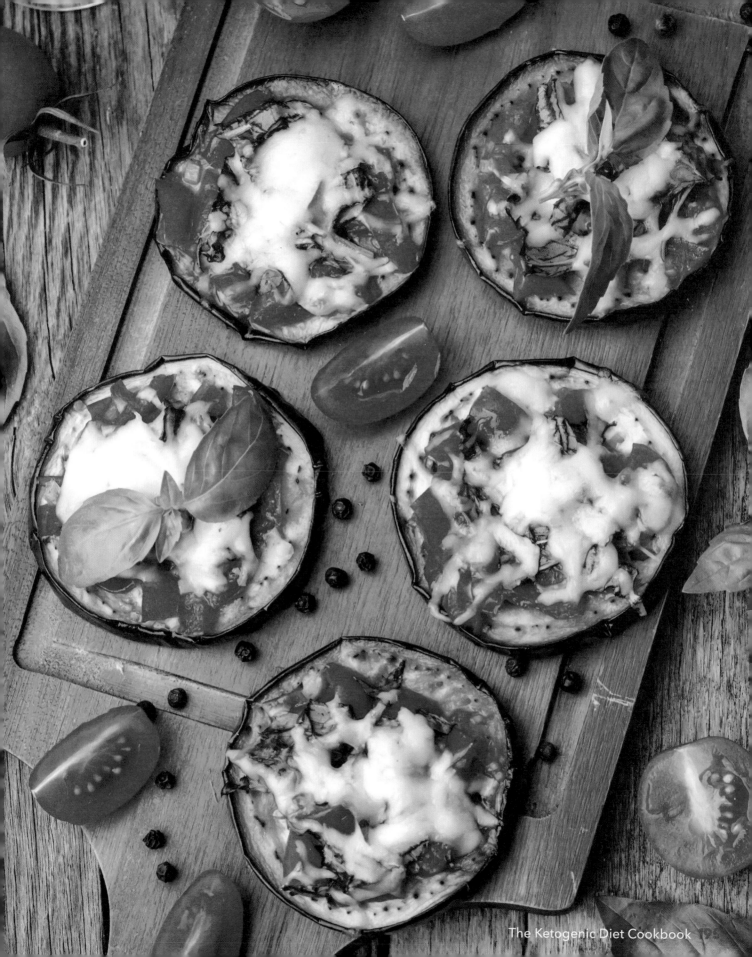

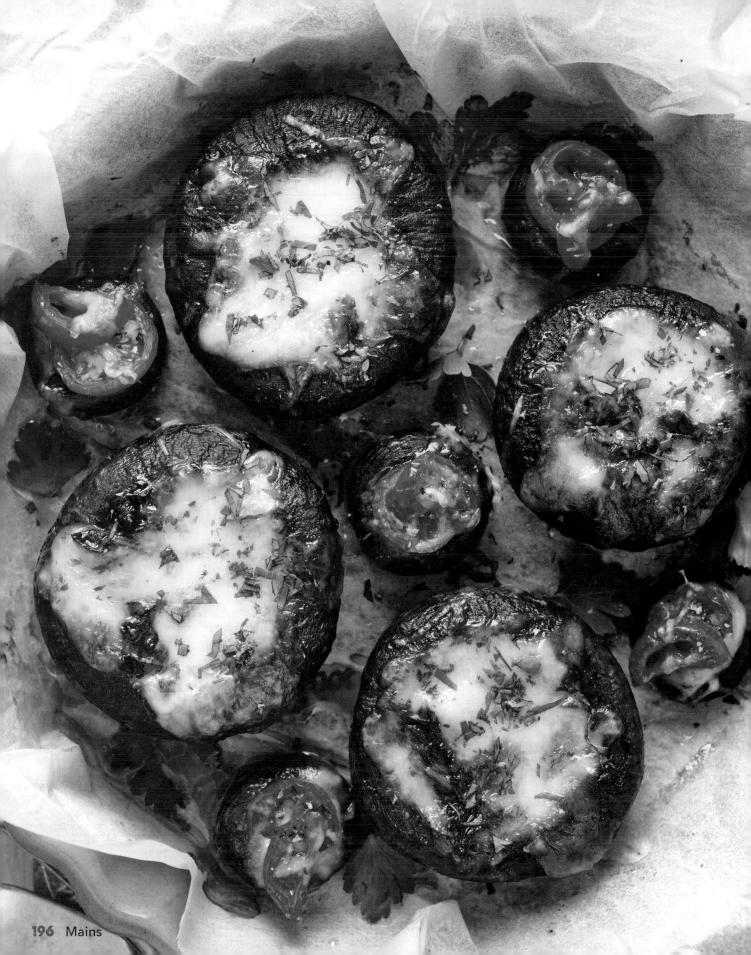

GRILLED PORTOBELLO "PIZZAS"

SERVES: 4 / CALORIES: 399 / FAT: 32G / NET CARBS: 7G / PROTEIN: 24G

8 large portobello mushroom caps, stems removed

¼ cup extra-virgin olive oil

4 cloves garlic, minced

2 tablespoons balsamic vinegar

1 cup tomato sauce

8 ounces mozzarella cheese, grated

4 ounces parmesan cheese, grated

Fresh basil leaves

1. In a large resealable bag, mix together extra-virgin olive oil and garlic. Once you've combined the mixture, place the mushroom caps in the bag and let them marinate for 1 hour.

2. After the caps have marinated, fill them with about ¼ cup of tomato sauce and top with freshly grated mozzarella. Top them with Parmesan.

3. Preheat grill to medium heat and place the caps on the grill for about 10 minutes, or until cheese melts. Remove from heat, top with torn basil leaves and serve.

BIG TIP

ADD MEAT! Top the mushrooms with ⅓ cup of pepperoni slices to enhance the savory flavor.
GO PALEO! Remove the cheese and replace with a paleo cheese from the supermarket.

DESSERTS

Who said you can't have dessert on keto? Sure, sugar is off limits, but sub in with a sweetener of your choice—from stevia to erythritol—and a whole new world opens up for you. If you're a chocoholic and can't keep away from the stuff, good news! You don't have to. Chocolate that's darker than 85% is actually allowed on keto in small amounts, and this is what goes into making keto-friendly desserts. And what desserts they are! A rich, decadent flourless cake that is the very essence of chocolate; a dense, squidgy almond flour and olive oil chocolate cake; a cheat's tiramisu that replaces sugary ladyfinger biscuits for a moist almond sponge; a berry-swirl cheesecake that brings home summer in any weather; an indulgent and versatile panna cotta…

Of course, a sweet tooth is a fickle thing; it strikes at most inopportune moments, when you may not necessarily have the time to make an extravagant dessert. Sometimes, it demands just that little sweet hit after dinner. For those moments, we have mug cakes. Using four ingredients or less, and coming together in mere minutes, it's the answer to all your dessert prayers on keto and endlessly customisable. So, the next time time someone says you can't eat dessert on a diet, show them that on keto, you can have your cake, and eat it too!

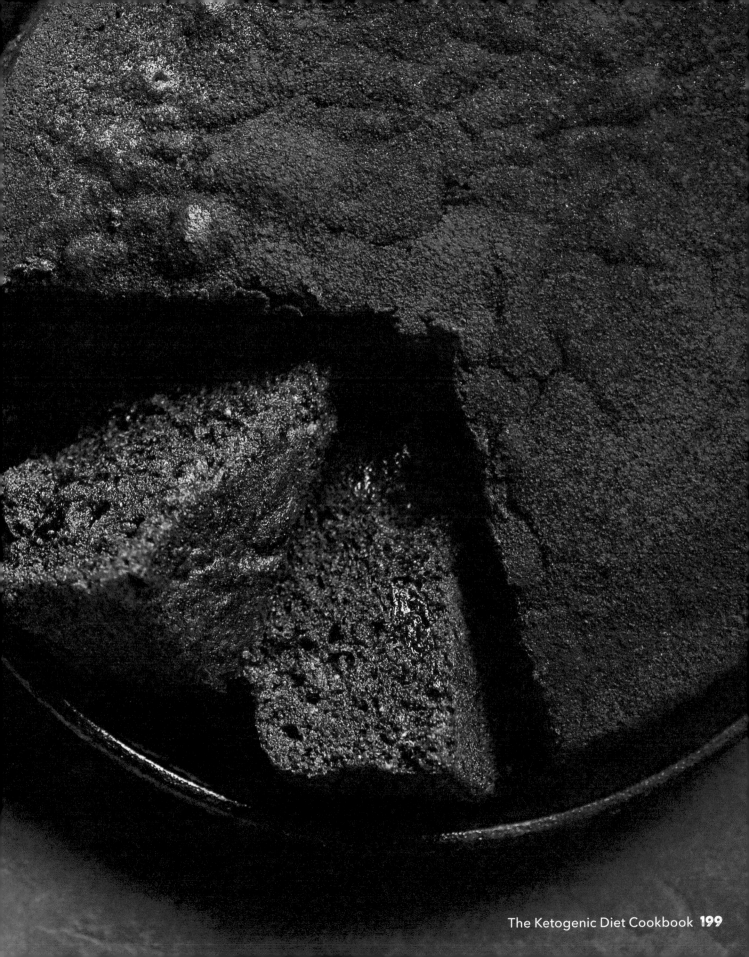

FLOURLESS CHOCOLATE CAKE

SERVES: 8 / CALORIES: 300 / FAT: 27G / NET CARBS: 6G / PROTEIN: 6G

7oz dark chocolate (85% or higher)

3.5 oz / ½ cup butter, cubed

½ cup heavy cream

4 eggs, separated

4 tablespoons Truvia or equivalent no-carb sweetener

1. Butter an 8' cake tin well.

2. Break the chocolate into even pieces and add to a bowl.

3. Add the butter and microwave in short bursts till the chocolate is melted. You can also do this over a double boiler.

4. Add the cream and Truvia and mix thoroughly. Taste the mix once to ensure the sweetness is to your liking.

5. Add the egg yolks, one at a time, mixing until just combined.

6. Whisk the egg whites in a separate bowl, with a pinch of salt, just until stiff peaks form (careful, do not over beat).

7. Fold the egg whites into the chocolate mixture in thirds, gently, until no white streaks remain.

8. Bake at 160°C (325°F) for about 45 minutes or until the rest of the cake is set, but the center just jiggles.

9. Cool to room temperature, then chill for at least 4 hours before serving. This also freezes really well.

BIG TIP

If you're a chocolate lover, this dessert is the ultimate tribute to all things cocoa – it's rich, dark, practically a truffle in cake form. Top it with a dollop of sweetened whipped cream for added indulgence.

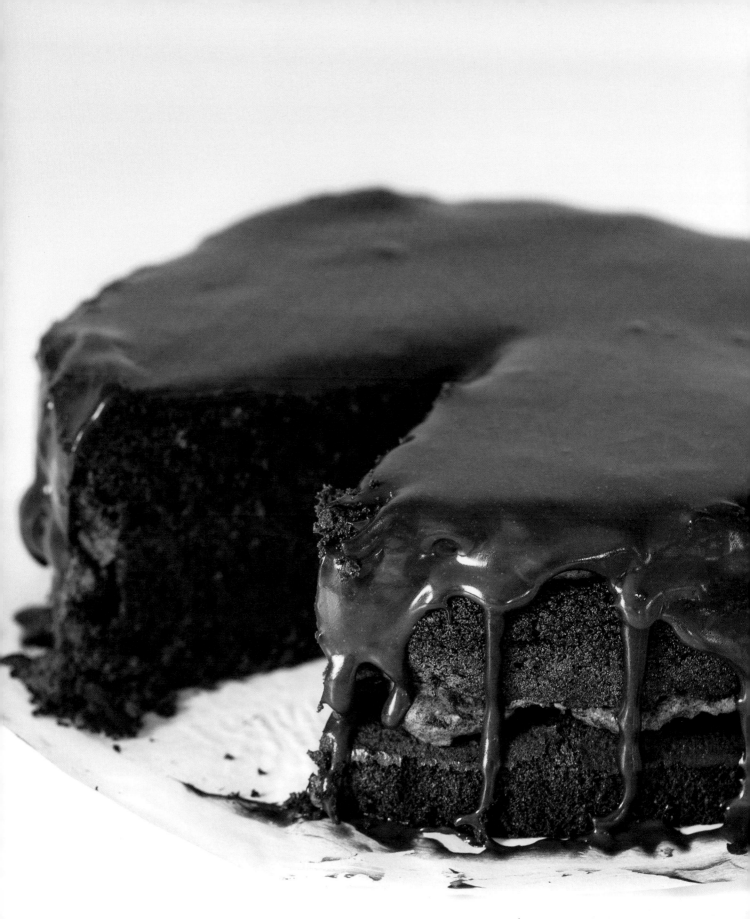

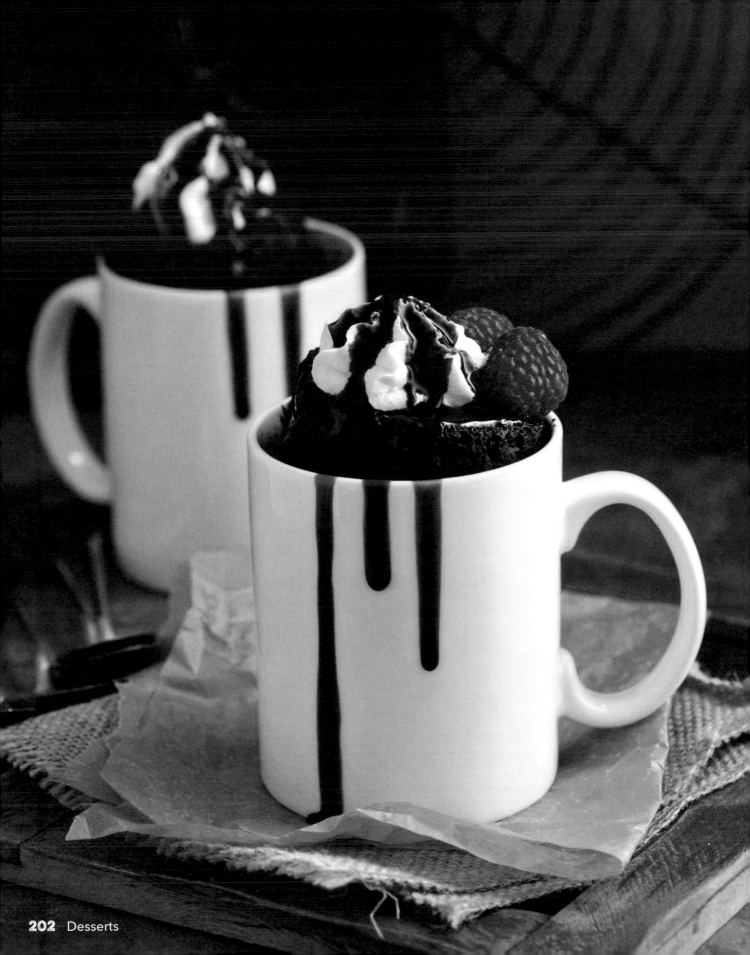

MICROWAVE CHOCOLATE CAKE
WITH CHOCOLATE GANACHE

SERVES: 1 / CALORIES: 175 / FAT: 18G / NET CARBS: 2G / PROTEIN: 1G

FOR THE MUG CAKE

¼ cup almond flour

2 tablespoons cocoa powder

Pinch of salt

1 tablespoon melted butter/coconut oil

1 tablespoon cream

A few drops of Stevia, to taste

A few drops of vanilla extract

1 egg

1. Whisk wet ingredients together in a mug, or a ramekin.

2. Add almond flour and cocoa powder to the wet ingredients and whisk until smooth.

3. Microwave for 1 minute for a fudgy texture, 1 minute 10 seconds for a more cakey texture.

4. Serve with our chocolate ganache, peanut butter or even whipped cream.

FOR THE GANACHE

1 square (.35oz) 90% Lindt Chocolate

1 tablespoon butter

1 tablespoon whipping cream

Stevia to taste

A tiny pinch of salt (if the butter is unsalted)

1. Break the chocolate into pieces and melt with butter in the microwave for 20 seconds.

2. Add in the cream and mix well.

3. Use as a topping where desired. Preferably on that microwave mug cake.

CHOCOLATE MOUSSE

SERVES: 4 / CALORIES: 239 / FAT: 22G / NET CARBS: 2G / PROTEIN: 3G

3.5 oz dark chocolate 85%

1 tablespoon salted butter (or unsalted butter + pinch of salt)

1 tablespoon cocoa powder

1 cup whipping cream

Stevia to taste

1. Melt the chocolate and butter in the microwave (about 30 seconds) in a bowl and mix together.

2. Whip together cream, cocoa powder and Stevia.

3. Add in the chocolate and butter to the cream mixture.

4. Whisk the mix well till soft peaks are formed and scoop into your serving dishes.

5. Refrigerate for at least 1 hour. Serve chilled.

BIG TIP

This is the easiest chocolate mousse you've ever made, but with all the richness of traditional mousse and none of the carbs.

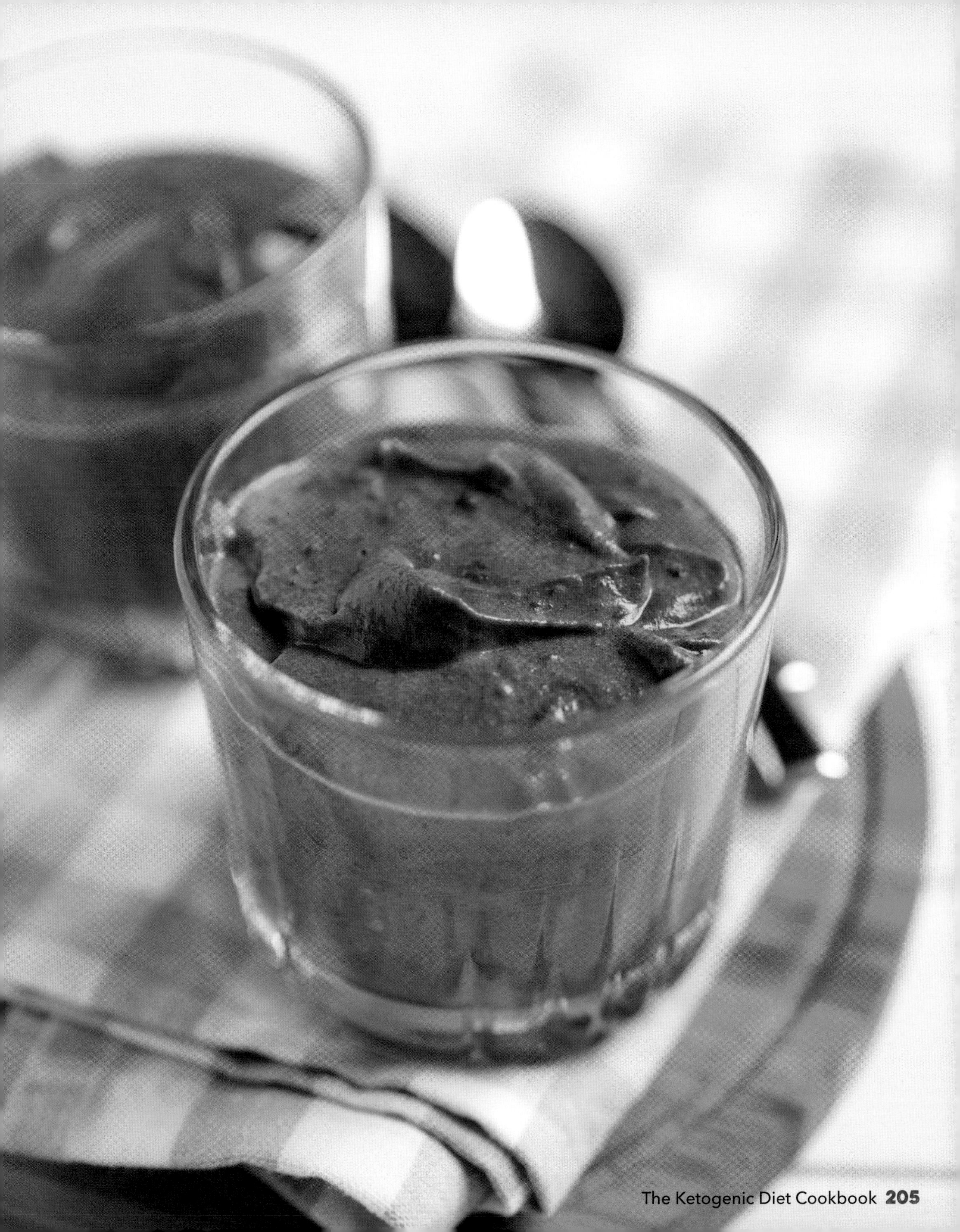

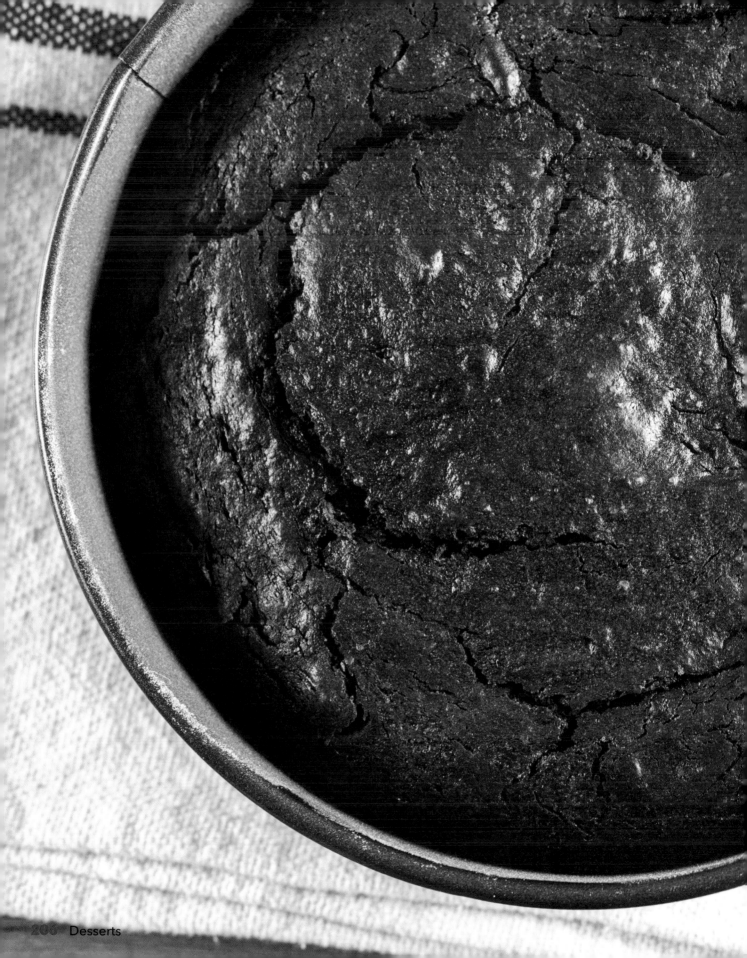

ALMOND FLOUR CHOCOLATE CAKE

SERVES: 8 / CALORIES: 323 / NET CARBS: 3G / FAT: 31G / PROTEIN: 8G

⅔ cup regular olive oil
(plus more for greasing)

3 tablespoons good-quality
cocoa powder (sifted)

⅔ cup boiling water

2 teaspoons vanilla extract

1½ cups almond flour

½ teaspoon baking soda

A pinch of salt

Stevia to taste

3 large eggs

1. Preheat your oven to 170°C or 340°F. Grease an 8-inch springform pan with a little oil and line the base with baking parchment.

2. Measure out the cocoa and whisk it into the boiling water until you have a smooth chocolate paste. Add in the vanilla extract, mix and set aside to cool.

3. In another bowl, combine the almond flour, baking soda and salt well.

4. Using an electric whisk, or a stand mixer, whisk together the olive oil, eggs and sweetener for about three minutes, until it becomes pale and frothy. Add in the cocoa mixture and whisk until well blended. Slowly tip in the almond flour and mix until everything is combined.

5. Pour into the cake tin and bake for about 30 minutes. You don't want to overbake this cake, because it can become dry and crumbly, so start testing it at the 25 minute mark—a toothpick inserted into the center should come out mostly clean but with a few crumbs attached.

6. Let it cool for about 10 minutes, then eat it while it's still warm, or let it cool all the way through and serve topped with some sweetened whipped cream.

BIG TIP

If you're hankering after a more traditional chocolate cake, this fits the bill perfectly. Almond flour gives it heft and olive oil pairs perfectly with the chocolate to make a moist, rich dessert that's perfect for any occasion like a birthday or an anniversary or even just your Sunday night dinner party.

TIRAMISU

SERVES: 8 / CALORIES: 308 / FAT: 29G / NET CARBS: 5G / PROTEIN: 16G

KETO MICROWAVE MUG BREAD

2 tbsp almond flour
1 tbsp butter
½ tsp baking powder
1 egg
½ tsp vanilla essence
Stevia to taste

TIRAMISU INGREDIENTS

14 oz mascarpone cheese
1 egg (separated)
2 tbsp cocoa powder (unsweetened)
Stevia/sweetener of your choice to taste
¼ cup fresh brewed espresso
2 tbsp whiskey
2 tbsp heavy cream
2 portions Keto Microwave Mug Bread

KETO MICROWAVE MUG BREAD

1. Mix all the ingredients together in a mug (or bowl).

2. Microwave the mug or bowl for 90 seconds.

3. Overturn the mug and the bread should slide out.

4. Slice the bread into discs or strips to use in the tiramisu.

TIRAMISU

1. Mix the espresso, whiskey and cream to make the soaking liquid.

2. Whisk the egg white to stiff peaks.

3. Whisk the yolk along with the powdered sweetener till it turns a pale yellow.

4. Add in the mascarpone cheese and 60 ml of the soaking liquid and whisk.

5. Fold in the egg white in two batches into the tiramisu cream mixture. Set aside.

6. Dip the sliced keto bread in the soaking liquid until soaked through, and use it to layer the bottom of you dish (or individual ramekins if using).

7. Pour the mascarpone cream mix over the bread and refrigerate until set.

8. Dust with cocoa powder before serving.

BIG TIP

If you love the classic Italian tiramisu, then you will love this buff-tinted low carb version. As a bonus, there's even a recipe for two-minute microwave keto bread!

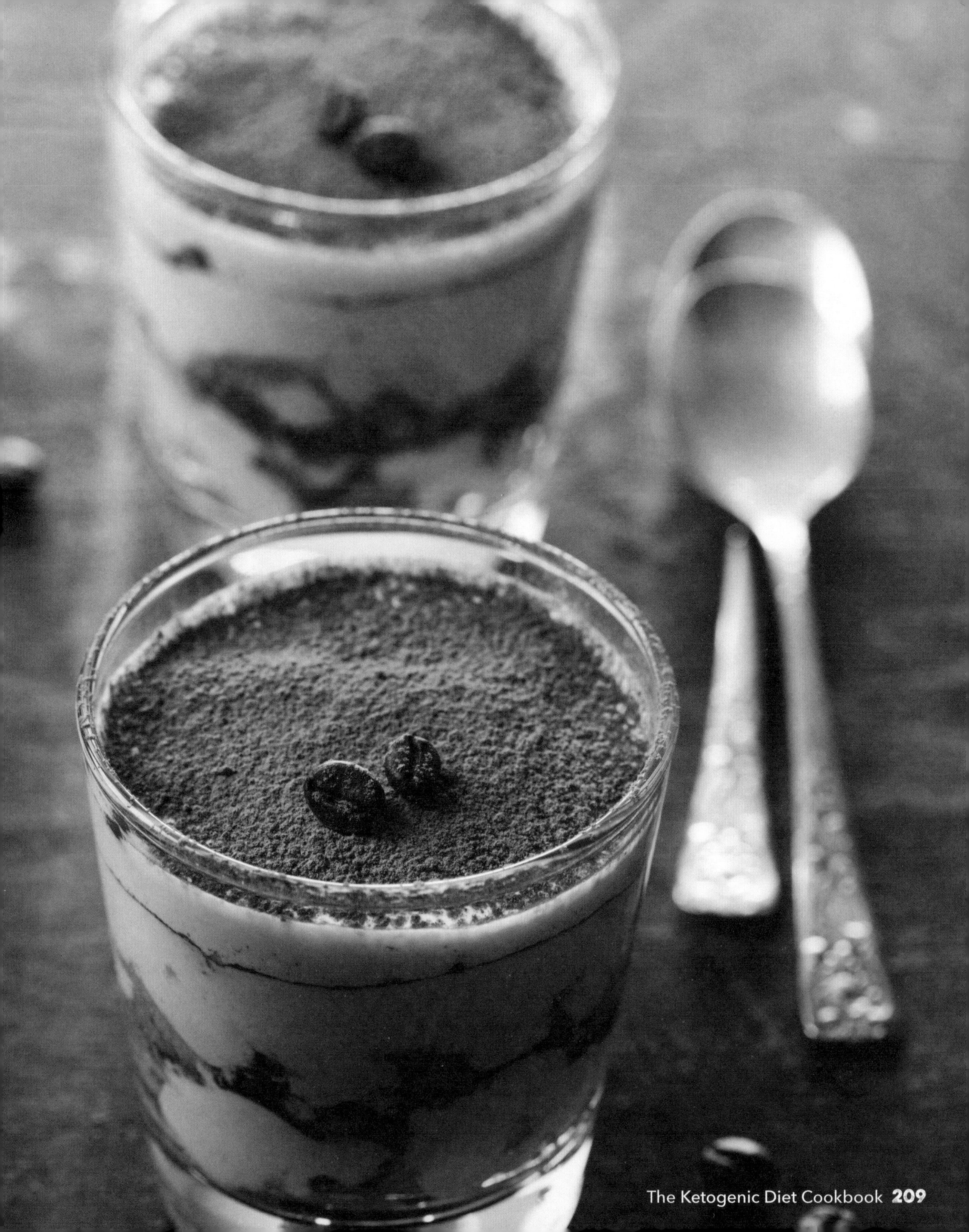

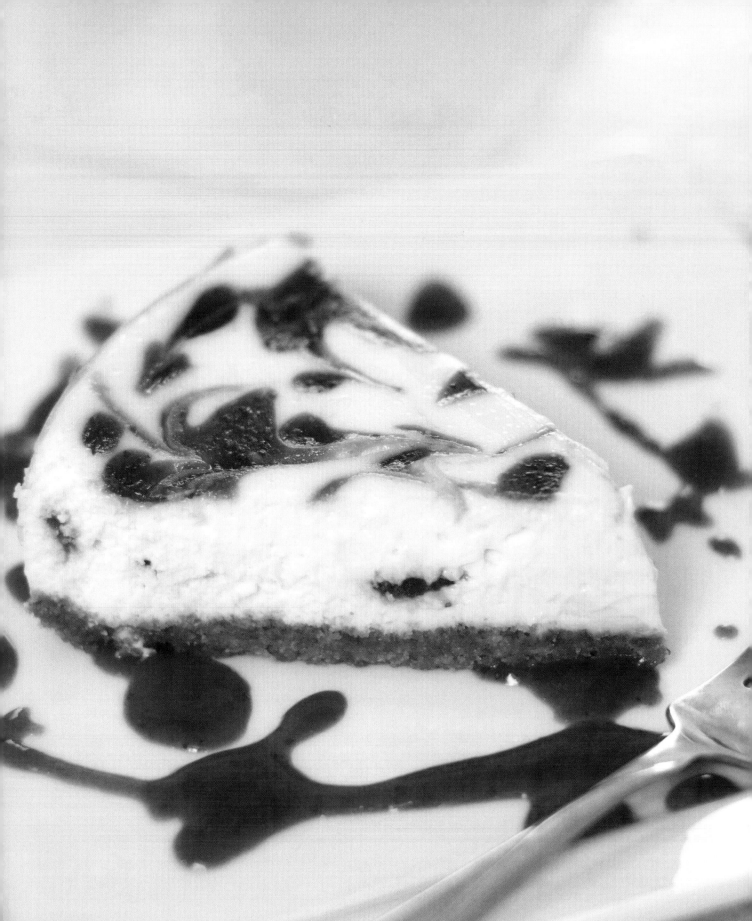

BERRY SWIRL CHEESECAKE

SERVES: 8 / CALORIES: 301 / FAT: 28G / NET CARBS: 5G / PROTEIN: 7G

FOR THE PUREE INGREDIENTS

7oz fresh berries or frozen berries
(Strawberries, raspberries or blueberries)

½ tbsp granulated sweetener or to taste

A pinch of salt

FOR THE BASE INGREDIENTS

1 cup almond flour

1.75oz / ¼ cup butter, melted

½ tbsp granulated sweetener
(or to taste)

Pinch of salt

FOR THE FILLING INGREDIENTS

8oz. cream cheese at room temperature

7 oz mascarpone at room temperature

2 eggs at room temperature

Juice of one lemon/lime

1 tbsp granulated sweetener (or to taste)

½ tsp vanilla extract

STEP 1

1. Throw the berries into a blender and puree as finely as possible.

2. Pass it through a sieve to get rid of all the seeds, then put it in a saucepan on a low flame.

3. Add the sweetener, and allow the mixture to reduce until it's a thick, jammy consistency. Put aside to cool.

STEP 2

1. Preheat the oven to 175°C/350°F. Line an 8 inch cake tin with parchment paper and grease thoroughly with butter.

2. In a bowl, add the almond flour, sweetener and salt and give it all a good mix.

3. Stir the melted butter into the flour and mix till it comes together like dough.

4. Press the almond flour mix into the cake tin and level it using your fingers, or a spoon.

5. Bake the base for 10 minutes, then take it out and leave it to cool.

STEP 3

1. Turn the oven down to 160°C/325°F.

2. Add the cream cheese and mascarpone to a bowl, along with the sweetener. Whisk it all together until it's smooth and lump free. Be careful not to whisk it too much, or it may cause the cheesecake to crack later (It's also important to have all the filling ingredients at room temperature to minimize the chance of the cheesecake cracking).

3. Add the lemon juice and whisk until just combined. Add the eggs one at a time, and again, whisk until it's just incorporated.

4. Add the vanilla, whisk, and taste test to make sure the sweetness is fine.

5. Divide the cheesecake filling into two parts. Stir the berry puree into one part. Then, alternating the two, spoon one ladle of the vanilla mix to the centre of your cake pan, then one of the berry. Do this until you've used up both batters (you should have concentric rings of batter).

6. Shake very lightly to level, then bake for 35 to 40 minutes, or until the sides are set but the center still has a bit of a jiggle.

7. Leave it to cool to room temperature on a rack, then chill it in the fridge for at least four hours.

CHOCOLATE PEANUT BUTTER MUG CAKE

SERVES: 1 PERSON / CALORIES: 533 / FAT: 47G / NET CARBS: 9G / PROTEIN: 21G

3 tbsp peanut butter

1 egg

1 tbsp cocoa butter (Can also be subbed with regular butter)

1 tbsp heavy cream

2 tbsp unsweetened cocoa powder

½ tsp baking powder

Stevia to taste

Whipped cream for topping

1. Mix together the peanut butter, cocoa powder, cocoa butter, egg, heavy cream, baking powder and stevia. Whisk till smooth.

2. Pour into mug.

3. Microwave for 1 minute.

4. Top with whipped cream.

5. Enjoy!

BIG TIP

This classic combination (peanut butter cups, anyone?) in cake form is a treat everyone will love. Plus, it's super easy to make and totally hits the spot when you're craving a sweet hit post dinner.

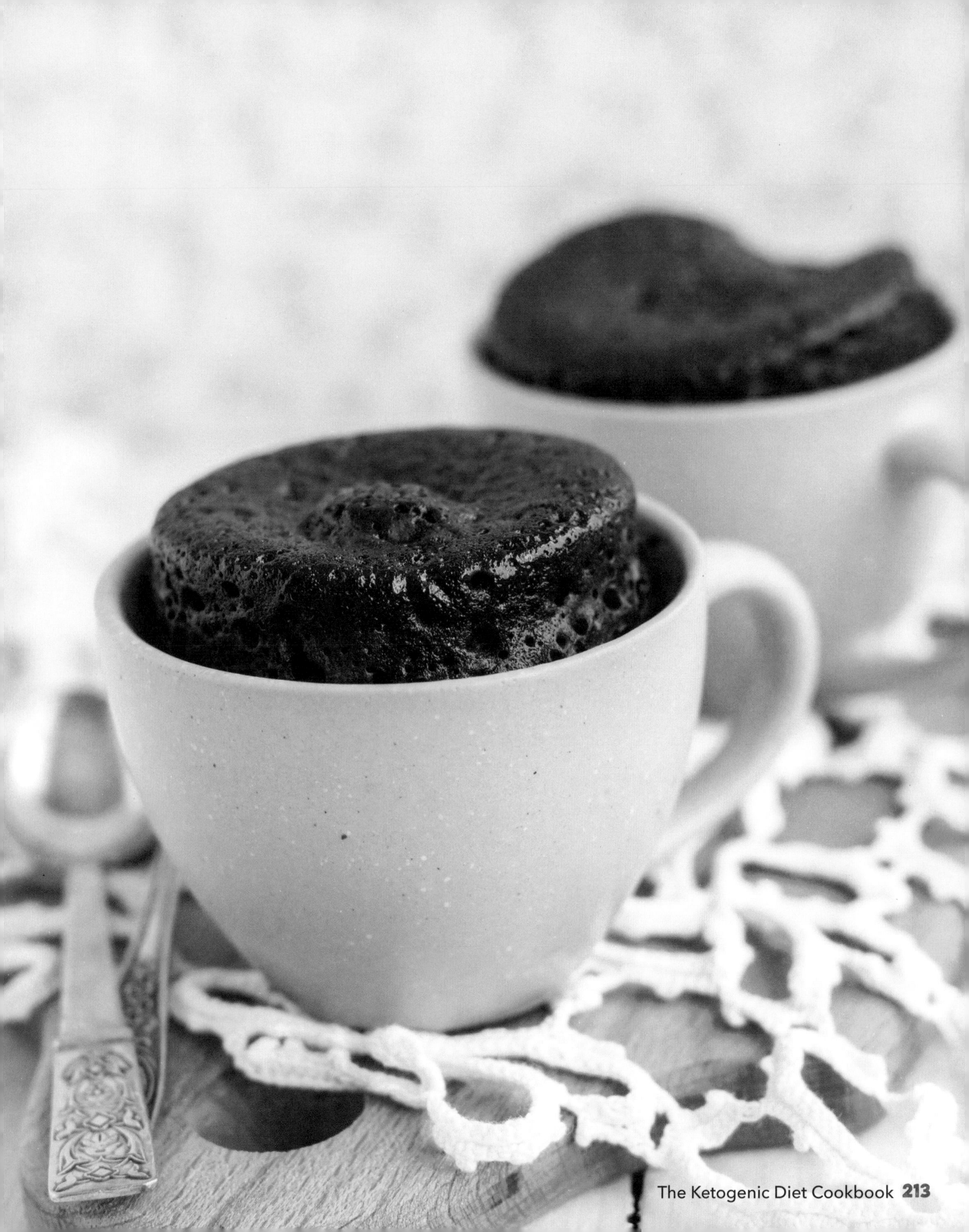

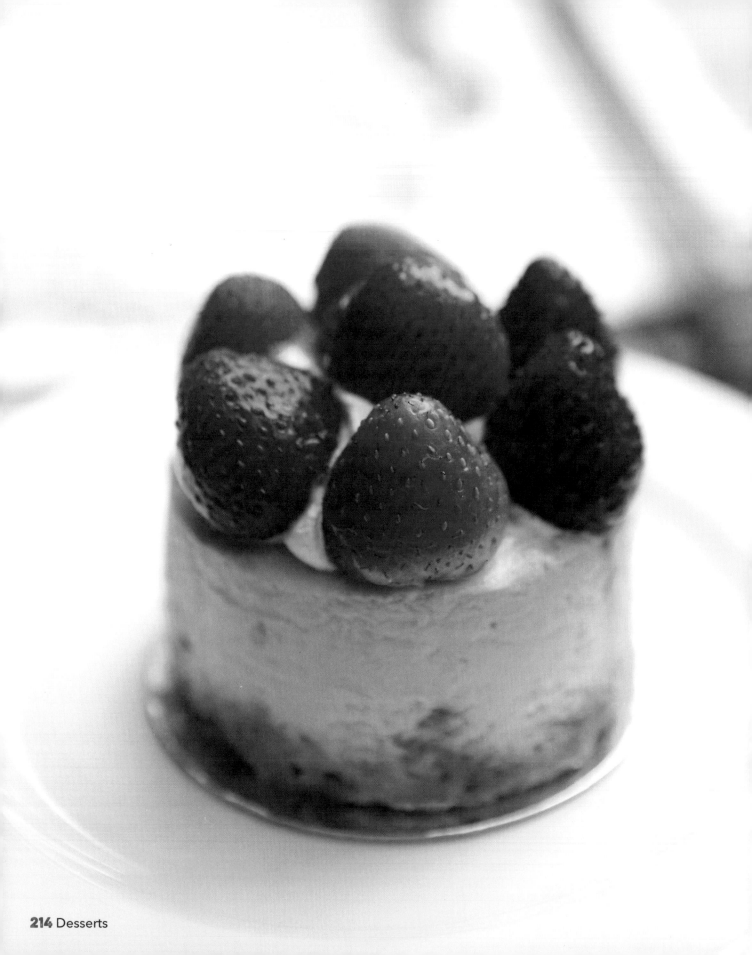

LEMON CHEESECAKE WITH FRESH STRAWBERRIES

SERVES 8 PEOPLE / CALORIES: 280 / FAT: 26G / NET CARBS: 1G / PROTEIN: 6G

1 cup desiccated coconut

½ cup almond flour or almond meal

1.75 oz / ¼ cup butter

Stevia to taste

8 oz grams cream cheese

½ cup yogurt

1 egg

Lemon juice to taste

Strawberries for garnish

1. For the base, melt the butter, add it to the almond flour and dessicated coconut. Mix together and press into the baking moulds as a base. Chill in the refrigerator for 10-15 minutes.

2. Mix the cream cheese, egg, yogurt, stevia, lemon juice together for the cheesecake.

3. Pour into the moulds.

4. Bake for about 10 minutes at 170°C/340°F till it stops jiggling when you give it a gentle shake.

5. Take it out, let it cool to room temperature, then chill for 4 hours.

6. Garnish with fresh strawberries.

BIG TIP

Delicious lemon cheese cakes that are bright and refreshing and a great way to break the monotony of chocolate-heavy desserts. You can make this in individual molds or turn into one single cheesecake.

INSTANT COCONUT FLOUR VANILLA CAKE

WITH CHOCOLATE PEANUTBUTTER GANACHE

SERVES: 1 / CALORIES: 212 / FAT: 42G / NET CARBS: 2G / PROTEIN: 6G

MUG CAKE INGREDIENTS
2 tbsp coconut flour
2 tbsp butter
2 tbsp coconut milk
½ tsp vanilla extract
¼ tsp baking powder
1 egg
Stevia to taste
A pinch of salt

1. Mix all the ingredients well in a bowl or in a mug.
2. Microwave for 90 seconds.
3. Serve.

CHOCOLATE GANACHE INGREDIENTS
1 tbsp butter or cocoa butter
1 tbsp peanut butter
1 tbsp unsweetened coco powder
1 tbsp coconut milk
Stevia to taste

1. Microwave the cocoa butter and peanut butter for 1 minute and mix till melted.
2. Add in the cocoa powder and stevia and mix well.
3. Add in the coconut milk and mix.
4. Serve.

BIG TIP

A delicious instant vanilla sponge made with coconut flour and topped with the classic chocolate and peanut butter flavoured ganache.

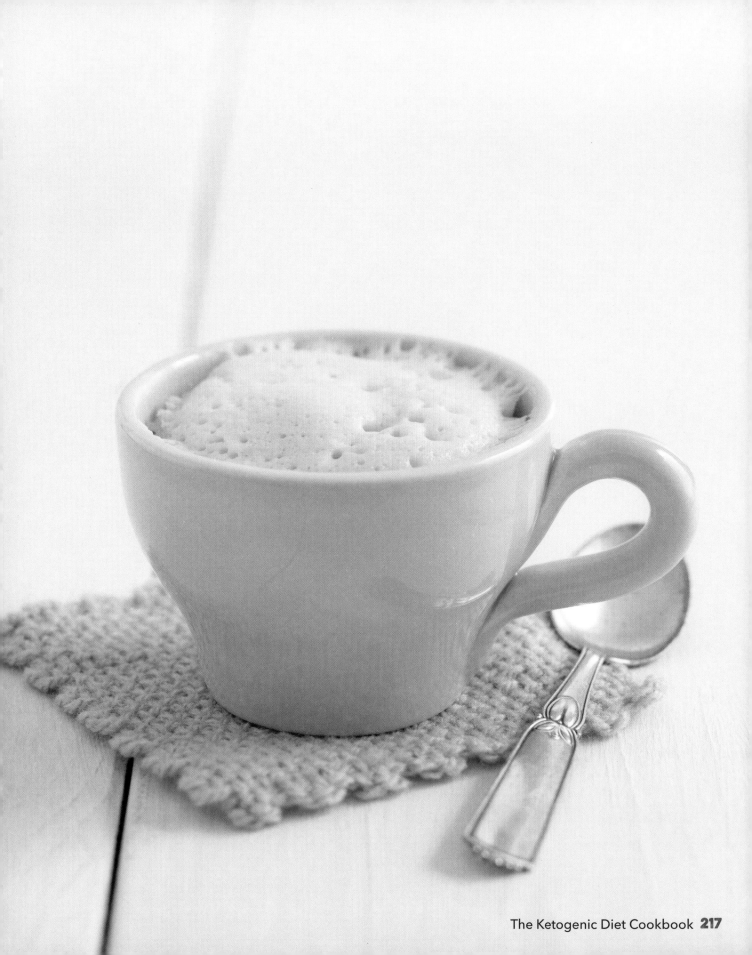

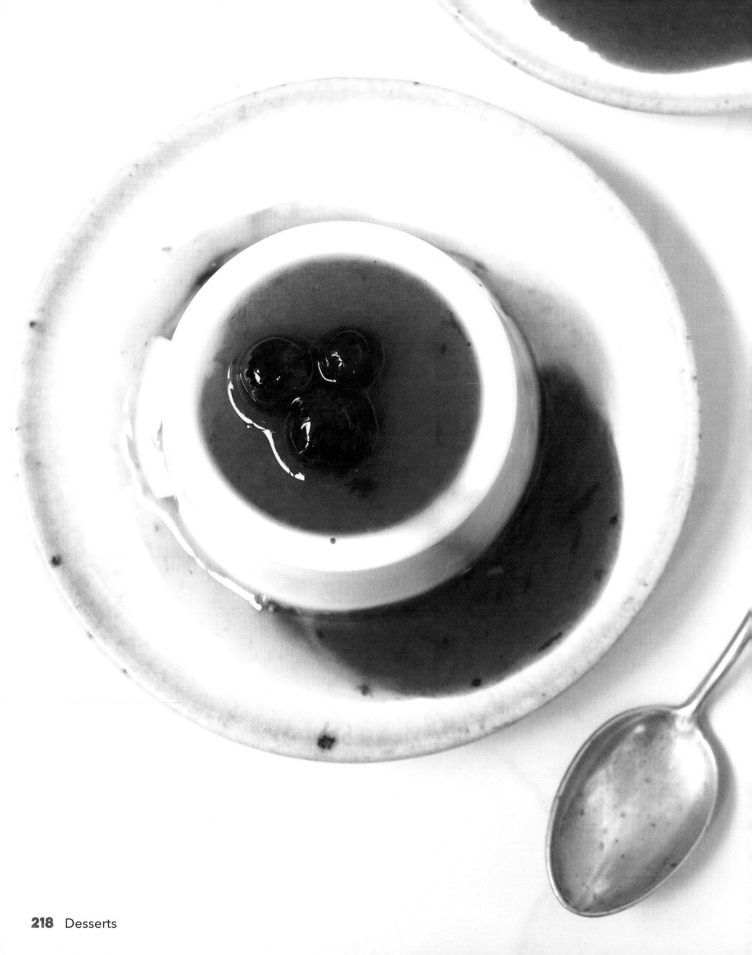

PANNA COTTA

SERVES: 3 / CALORIES: 204 / FAT: 20G / NET CARBS: 3G / PROTEIN: 3G

1 cup light cream (25-30% fat)
(or heavy cream for a creamier
panna cotta)

1 spare teaspoon gelatin

1 vanilla pod, or 1 teaspoon vanilla
extract

Stevia or preferred sweetener to taste

1. Add the gelatin to two tablespoons of water and set aside for five minutes to allow it to "bloom."

2. Pour the cream into a small saucepan and set it on low heat.

3. Slit the vanilla pod lengthwise down the center.

4. Using the tip of the knife, scrape the seeds from the pod and add them to the cream.

5. Add the pod to the cream as well (If you're using vanilla extract, add it to the cream once you take it off the heat).

6. Once the cream begins to just simmer, take it off the heat. Discard the vanilla pod. Add the gelatin to the cream and mix well until it's completely dissolved and no lumps remain.

7. Pour into moulds and leave to set in the fridge for at least 4 hours.

8. To make coffee panna cotta, add a teaspoon of instant coffee granules to each mould and stir it into the hot cream.

9. To unmould the panna cotta, dip the moulds briefly in a bowl of hot water, then upend it on a plate. Serve the vanilla panna cotta topped with mixed berries.

BIG TIP

You won't believe how easily this panna cotta comes together, and
how versatile it is. Feel free to play around with the flavors too!

INDEX

ABOUT THE
AUTHOR

Sahil Makhija is the frontman of one of India's most popular metal bands, but the keto community know him best for Headbanger's Kitchen, his youtube channel and show, which has been making keto easy and achievable for thousands across the world. He's been an avid food lover since he was a child, and has been cooking for friends and family since the age of 12, which possibly explains why he needed the diet later in life. He even aspired to be a chef, until he discovered his love for heavy metal music. Today, Headbanger's Kitchen is an easy amalgam of his two passions—metal and food—in an unexpected, but always delicious pairing.

He can be found on youtube.com/HeadbangersKitchen or instagram @headbangerskitchen, or check out his website at headbangerskitchen.com

ACKNOWLEDGMENTS

This cookbook has been a pleasure to work on and something I wouldn't have been able to do had Cider Mill Press not shown this faith in me. My heartfelt thanks to John Whalen, Brittany Wason, Cindy Butler, Rayna Knight, Annalisa Sheldahl, and the entire team at Cider Mill Press for giving this incredible opportunity. I could not have done this without the help of my wife Deepti Unni, both my greatest support and most discerning critic.

ABOUT CIDER MILL PRESS BOOK PUBLISHERS

Good ideas ripen with time. From seed to harvest, Cider Mill Press brings fine reading, information, and entertainment together between the covers of its creatively crafted books.
Our Cider Mill bears fruit twice a year, publishing a new crop of titles each spring and fall.

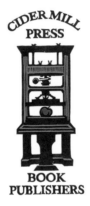

"Where Good Books Are Ready for Press"

Visit us online:
cidermillpress.com

or write to us at
PO Box 454
12 Spring St.
Kennebunkport, Maine 04046

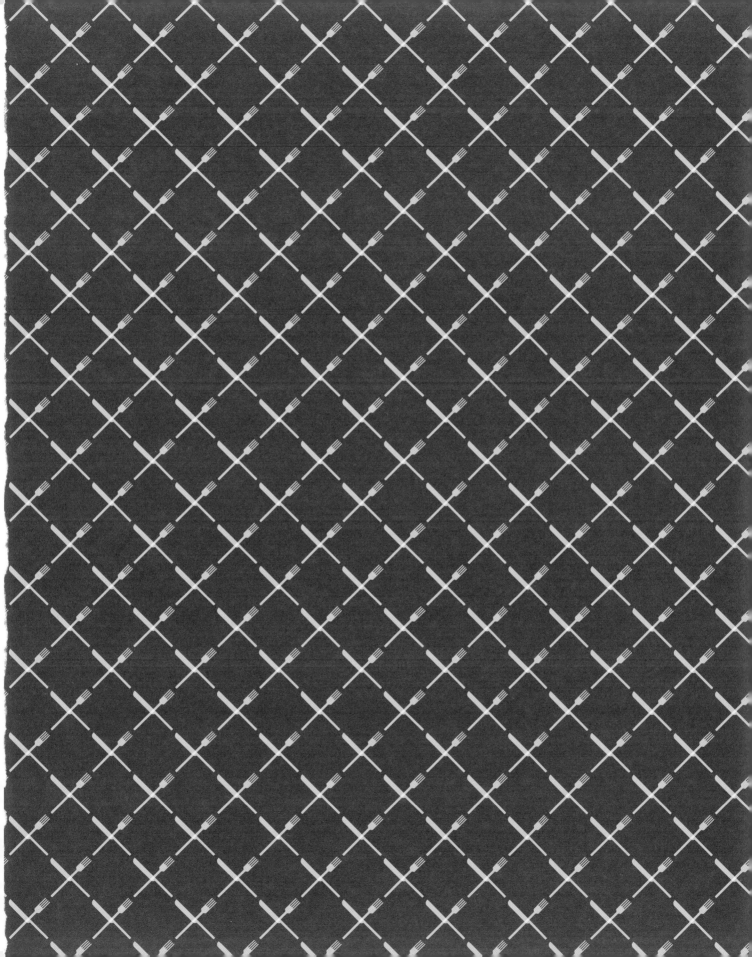

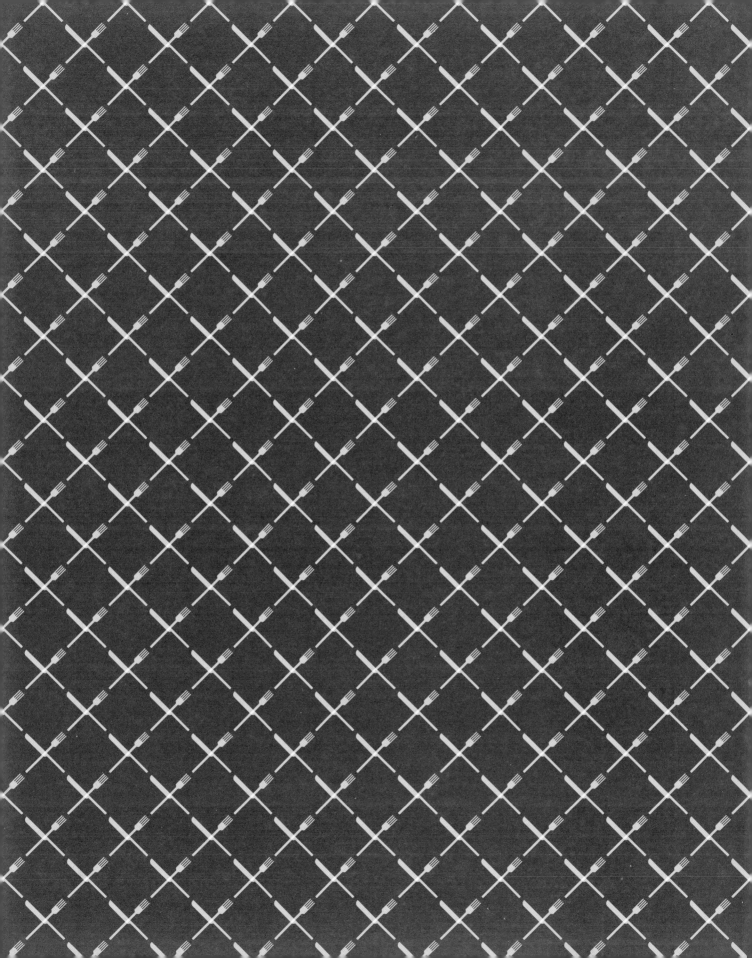